A to Z Guideline Manual in

NURSING

Performance Evaluation Tool

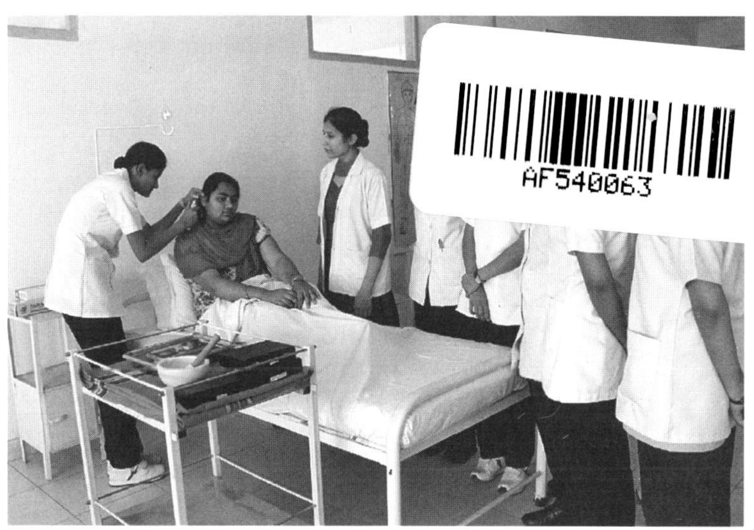

A to Z Guideline Manual in NURSING Performance Evaluation Tool

(for Practitioners and Students)

SN Nanjunde Gowda MSc (N) DPN PhD
Professor and Principal
Anil Baghi College of Nursing
Ferozepur, Punjab, India
Formerly, Principal
Padmashree College of Nursing
Ikon Nursing College
Dayananda Sagar Nursing College
Bengaluru, Karnataka, India

Jyothi Nanjunde Gowda MSc (N) DPN
Vice-Principal
Anil Baghi College of Nursing
Ferozepur, Punjab, India

Foreword
BN Muninarayanappa

JAYPEE *The Health Sciences Publisher*
New Delhi | London | Philadelphia | Panama

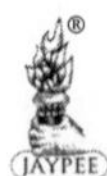

Jaypee Brothers Medical Publishers (P) Ltd

Headquarters

Jaypee Brothers Medical Publishers (P) Ltd
4838/24, Ansari Road, Daryaganj
New Delhi 110 002, India
Phone: +91-11-43574357
Fax: +91-11-43574314
Email: jaypee@jaypeebrothers.com

Overseas Offices

J.P. Medical Ltd
83 Victoria Street, London
SW1H 0HW (UK)
Phone: +44-2031708910
Fax: +02-03-0086180
Email: info@jpmedpub.com

Jaypee-Highlights Medical Publishers Inc
City of Knowledge, Bld. 237, Clayton
Panama City, Panama
Phone: +1 507-301-0496
Fax: +1 507-301-0499
Email: cservice@jphmedical.com

Jaypee Medical Inc
325 Chestnut Street
Suite 412, Philadelphia, PA 19106, USA
Phone: +1 267-519-9789
Email: jpmed.us@gmail.com

Jaypee Brothers Medical Publishers (P) Ltd
17/1-B Babar Road, Block-B, Shaymali
Mohammadpur, Dhaka-1207
Bangladesh
Mobile: +08801912003485
Email: jaypeedhaka@gmail.com

Jaypee Brothers Medical Publishers (P) Ltd
Bhotahity, Kathmandu, Nepal
Phone: +977-9741283608
Email: kathmandu@jaypeebrothers.com

Website: www.jaypeebrothers.com
Website: www.jaypeedigital.com

Inquiries for bulk sales may be solicited at: jaypee@jaypeebrothers.com

A to Z Guideline Manual in Nursing Performance Evaluation Tool

First Edition: **2016**

ISBN 978-93-5250-150-2

Printed at Rajkamal Electric Press, Plot No. 2, Phase-IV, Kundli, Haryana.

Dedicated to

Nurses of India
and
our colleagues and students
for contributing to our professional
growth and development

Contributors

Anupama Dayanand MSc (N)
Associate Professor
Anil Baghi College of Nursing
Ferozepur, Punjab, India

Devi Nanjappa MSc (N)
Principal
Smt Nagarathnamma College of Nursing
Bengaluru, Karnataka, India

Kanwalpreet Kaur MSc (N)
Associate Professor
Anil Baghi College of Nursing
Ferozepur, Punjab, India

Lakshmamma VT MSc (N)
Principal
Kempe Gowda Institute of Nursing
Bengaluru, Karnataka, India

Lakshmi Devi MSc (N)
Principal
Global College of Nursing
Bengaluru, Karnataka, India

Linta Siby MSc (N)
Associate Professor
Anil Baghi College of Nursing
Ferozepur, Punjab, India

Rajni Siotra MSc (N)
Lecturer
Anil Baghi College of Nursing
Ferozepur, Punjab, India

Ramu MSc (N) PhD
Principal
Sreedevi College of Nursing
Tumkur, Karnataka, India

R Sree Raj Kumar MSc (N)
Associate Professor
College of Nursing
Adesh University
Bathinda, Punjab, India

Yatti Kumar Gowda MSc (N) PhD
Principal
Alva College of Nursing
Mudabidri, Karnataka, India

Foreword

The challenge of becoming a nurse has always been a considerable one. The work is often difficult emotionally and at times extremely hard physically. Over the years, nursing evolved through many forms and in recent years, it has become technically based and scientifically challenging.

Human beings are goal-directed creatures constantly striving for meaning, significances and purposes. We all need a role for something to work towards, to give us a sense of value and control. The authors of this book have used their clinical teaching, management and research expertise to bring out the contemporary and innovative thoughts practiced in Indian Nursing Institutes, Hospitals, and at the Department of Nursing, Ministry of Health, Sultanate of Oman. However, to implement the standard practices, the authors observed how to get new innovative thoughts into mind and how to get the old ones out.

I recommend this book to be used for the entire nursing program and should be on the book shelf of every student and practicing nurse today.

I congratulate the authors who brought together the most important ideas from the old and new *A to Z Guideline Manual in Nursing Performance Evaluation Tool* together.

BN Muninarayanappa
Registrar
Karnataka State Nursing Council
Bengaluru, Karnataka, India

Preface

A to Z Guideline Manual in Nursing Performance Evaluation Tool has been designed in many areas to explain the key steps which are necessary to perform nursing skills and provide cues to the critical thinking needed for client care.

The basics of nursing education depend on theory and clinical exposure. The quality of nursing education is only gained through theory and clinical experience. Nurse educators have the greater responsibilities to develop psychomotor and technical skills with the learner. If the theory and clinical experiences are systematically planned, organized and adhering to the criteria of evaluation, only then we can expect nursing care skills are imparted to the learner. The nursing educational institutes play a vital role in developing criteria for evaluating performance of learner and teacher.

In order to develop and provide high quality of care, it is necessary to develop appropriate standard of care and appropriate evaluation tool. Setting up standard is the first step in the evaluation process.

Two distinctive features of this book are the activities which one can get involved with, and evaluation of clinical practice behavior of learner at the desired level of performance.

SN Nanjunde Gowda
Jyothi Nanjunde Gowda

Preface

Acknowledgments

A special acknowledgment to all our colleagues, for their cooperation and encouragement, which we have received throughout the completion of this work.

Our sincere appreciation also goes to our fellow teachers and to all our students who have encouraged and participated in photographs and inspired us in making this book possible.

Our warm appreciation and thanks goes to Shri Jitendar P Vij (Group Chairman), Mr Ankit Vij (Group President) and Mr Tarun Duneja (Director–Publishing) of M/s Jaypee Brothers Medical Publishers (P) Ltd, New Delhi, India, for sharing our vision for this book and giving us the chance to turn vision into reality.

Above all, we are thankful to Almighty God, for bestowing His bountiful grace for successful completion of this book.

Contents

Florence Nightingale and Nursing

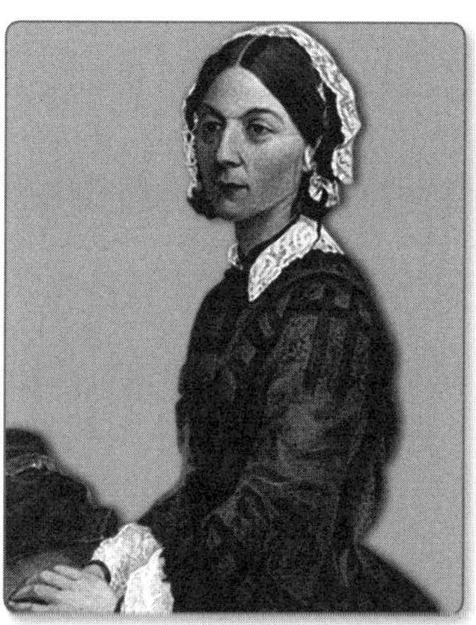

Florence Nightingale can hardly be considered a product of her time, since she was far ahead of and beyond it, but she found the time ripe for her genius as the founder of modern trained nursing.

While she was still little girl, she showed her kindness of heart and her wish to be helpful by nursing sick animals. At the age of nine, she often expressed a wish to be useful to sick persons. When she was in her teens, she visited among the sick poor of her neighborhood and did what she could do for them. Among her relatives, she was ready and competent.

Her Wish to be a Nurse

Soon after she was twenty, she asked her parents to permit her to go into a hospital and learn to be a nurse, so that she might care for the poor people of her own neighborhood. They knew something of the dreadful conditions existing in hospitals and could not bring their mind to the thought of their daughter doing such a thing. She would not go without their consent, and the situation grieved her greatly. She believed that an earnest life must express itself in work for humanity, and that "the service of man is the service of God". She longed for the chance to be helpful in a large way. She was always deeply religious. She once told her sister, "I look to thirty as the age when our savior took up his work. I am trying to prepare myself to follow in his foot-steps when I am as old as he was".

CHAPTER

1

Introduction to Evaluation Process

Introduction

Education technology refers to the development of various methods of educational technological inventions. These advances come from the interaction of changing concepts with changing techniques leading to new ways of performing educational activities.

Basic of nursing education depending on theory and clinical exposure. The quality of nursing education only gained through theory and clinical experience, nursing educators have the greater responsibilities to develop psychomotor and technical skills with the learner, if the theory and clinical experience systematically planned organized and adhering to the criteria of evaluation, only we can expect nursing care skills are imparted in the learner. The nursing educational institute play a vital role in developing criteria for evaluating performance of learner and teachers.

In order to develop and provide high quality of care, it is necessary to develop appropriate standards of care and appropriate evaluation tools. Setting up of standard is the first step in the evaluation process.

Evaluation process standards describe the behavior of learner at the desired levels of performance. This specifies the desired methods of specific nursing interventions. This involves all the activities concerned with delivering patient care. These standards measures the nursing actions or lack of actions involving patient care

Thus the process standard assist in measuring the degree of skills, with which a technique or procedure was carried out by the learner which includes the levels of learner and client interaction. This includes:

- Nursing techniques
- Nursing procedures
- Nursing activities (in terms of quality of care, appropriateness of care, adequacy of care
- Learner with appropriate assessment collects data, prioritize the needs, and identify the expected outcome and plan of care.

Objectives of Performance Evaluation

1. Provides reflective feedback on the work of learner and staff for a given period of time.
2. To acknowledge and encourage appropriate performance.

3. To identify and remove ineffective performance and behaviors.
4. To identify the areas of growth for the staff and as well as the organization.
5. To ensure quality care and to maintain high standards of care.
6. Performance of learner and staff is assessed in relation to the behaviorally stated work goals.
7. Observation of the representative sample of the learner and staff total work activities, should be taken into consideration.
8. When several areas of performance requires improvement ,indicate which area has the highest priority for improvement.
9. Purpose of the evaluation is to improve the work performance and job satisfaction.

Standards of Nursing Documentation

Introduction

Creating and maintaining records is an integral part of health care. Complete, accurate, relevant, and timely documentation is crucial for the continuity of patients care.

By maintaining proper standards of documentation, health care providers are honoring the expectation of the nursing profession.

As a nursing educator, learner or as a registered nurse or midwife, you are personally accountable for your practice and in the exercise of your professional accountability.

1. Act always in such a manner as to promote and safeguard the interests and well being of patients and clients.
2. Ensure that no addition or omission on your part or within the sphere of responsibility is detrimental to the interests, conditions or safety of patients and clients.

Purpose and Value of Documentation

Documentation of care is synonymous with care itself. If it is not documented, it has not been done. A well documented medical record must:

- Reflect patients care given
- Demonstrate the expected outcomes of treatment
- Help to plan and coordinate care contributed by each members of professional team
- Allow interdisciplinary exchange of information about the patient
- Provide evidence of the nurses' legal responsibilities towards the patient
- Demonstrate adherence to standards, rules, regulations, and laws of nursing and midwifery practice
- Provide information for analysis of cost benefit and reduction
- Reflect ethical and professional conduct and responsibility.

Guidelines for Nursing Documentation

1. Use only your institutions approved forms. Do not improvise and/or introduce new forms unless approved by your health institution.
2. All nursing documentation must be written in black or blue ink (including narcotics and blood transfusions).
3. Place the patient identification (sticker) on every page or record patient's identification on each page (full name, age, sex, hospital number, date of admission, ward, and bed number).
4. Use standard date at the beginning of each shift (day, month, and year).
5. Each entry must be authenticated (name, signature and title).
6. Unfinished documentation should be signed before starting a new page.
7. Do not leave blank space between entries.
8. Draw a line ending last sentence.
9. Do not erase and/or obliterate error. Draw a line through an error, write "Error", date and initialize.
10. Document omission as new entry.
11. Use only standard and institutions approved abbreviations, do not use short handwriting.
12. Do not alter previously documented patients records.
13. All nursing documentation must be ligible, relevant, accurate and concise (e.q. clear handwritinq).
14. Do not document using vague or broad statement, e.g. good day, bad food, adequate, slept well and good, satisfactory, etc.
15. Do not transcribe physician's orders.
16. Do not document interpreatation, what someone said, heard or smelled unless the information is crucial.
17. Use appropriate graphic and specialized flow sheet according to department's policy.
18. Check that you have the correct chart before you begin documenting.
19. Do not document care unless it has been provided.
20. Document explanations if care was not provided.
21. Do not document other nurse' care for patients.
22. Do not document care that was provided in previous shifts.
23. Do not duplicate entries.
24. The documentation must reflect the nursing process, initial assessment, reassessment, planning, implementation or nursing intervention, and evaluation of care provided. Record changes of patient's condition and complications.

Performance Evaluation in Nursing

Administration of Tool

1. The clinical assessment of fundamentals of nursing course based on a formal clinical assessment on each nursing procedures.
2. There are two major areas of student's performance being measured in a continuous assessment. Application of nursing process and professional conduct, each area identifies certain standards which must be met by the students in order to achieve the highest marks for that standard. The standard is the optimum behavior expected from the students. Form is provided to record the score of students' performance titled continuous assessment tool.
3. This clinical continuous assessment form is to be provided to the student at the beginning of the clinical experience in which it will be used.
4. The clinical teacher is to discuss student progress and clinical performance on a continuous basis. Strengths and weakness of the students to be identified and documented on anecdotal notes.
5. The clinical assessment form is to be completed by the clinical teacher at the end of the clinical experience.
6. The completed form is to be discussed with the student and an explanation provided for any marks that are not understood by the students.
7. The students' signature on the form only indicates that she/he has been presented with the form. If the student disagrees with the marking, the students should write a comment on the form to that effect and may pursue the matter with the division coordinator, if there is one, or with principal.

Use of the Tool (Example, Rating Scale)

1. **Each standard has a four point rating scale with the following definitions:**

Standard met	The student achieved all of the items identified in the standard.
Standard almost met	The student achieved more than half of the items identified in the standard.
Standard far from met	The student achieved less than half of the items identified in the standard.
Standard not met	The student did not achieved the items identified in the standard.

1. Each standard has different points depending on the importance of that standard to the overall assessment.

2. The score of the clinical assessment form enter the appropriate point in the box provided at the right side of the form against each standard.
3. Students must be informed when they are being graded for the final assessment.

NB: If a student misses any critical element he/she should be reassessed.

If you are using different scale student will be graded as per scale.

Guidelines for the Use of Clinical Continuous Assessment Tool

Guidelines are provided for the clinical teacher in order to increase the objectivity of the clinical continuous assessment and to maintain the standard among the entire nursing institute. Assessment should be based on knowledge and skills of the course objectives.

Guidelines (Nursing Process Approach)

I. **Assessment and Diagnosis**
   1. **Collects data about patients needs**
      a. Provides privacy, selects suitable time and place
      b. Collects relevant data such as personal family, medical history
      c. Identifies the deviations from health and illness and from normal to abnormal.
   2. **Identifies basic needs of the patients**
      a. Lists the basic needs, oxygen, nutrition, hygiene, elimination, comfort, rest, sleep, love and safety.
      b. Makes relevant observations, vital signs, and deviation from the physical examination.
      c. Identifies the actual problems—lack of oxygen, lack of comfort and rest, sleeplessness.
      d. Recognizes the potential problems such as injuries, chemical, mechanical and thermal problems.
   3. **Categorizes the patients' needs/problems**
      a. Categorizes the basic needs according to Maslow's hierarchy
      b. Categorizes the actual and potential problems
      c. Identifies the significance of the data collected.
   4. **Formulates nursing diagnosis**
      a. Organizes the data and utilizes teachers assistance in analyzing the data
      b. Identifies the significance of the data
      c. Makes nursing diagnosis at the basic level on the basis of data.

II. **Planning**

1. **Prioritizes the patients' needs**
   a. Establishes priority of needs on the basis of assessment made, resources available and urgency
   b. Identifies the clients values and beliefs and priorities
   c. Identifies the importance of providing care as per the priority of needs
   d. Organizes the nursing care plans by priority.
2. **States the outcome criteria**
   a. Derives the outcome criteria relating to the goals
   b. Describes the outcome criteria specific, observable and measurable responses of the patients
   c. Recognizes the importance of outcome criteria for evaluating care.
3. **Plans nursing action for each needs of the patients**
   a. Makes appropriate nursing care plans using the immediate and long-term nursing objectives
   b. Organizes nursing care plans using the investigations and medical orders
   c. Seek guidance from senior nursing staff when needed
   d. Identifies patients social background
   e. Recognizes the individuals needs and problems
   f. Considers the patients values/beliefs in planning care.
4. **Plans rationale for nursing action**
   a. Nursing actions are safe and appropriate for the individual's age, health and so on
   b. Recognizes it is achievable with the resources
   c. Congruent with clients values and beliefs
   d. Follows basic scientific principles in planning care.
5. **Formulates the needed patient health instructions**
   a. Identifies the felt needs and potential problems of the patient.
   b. Involves the patient, family members in planning care
   c. Utilizes appropriate time for teaching
   d. Seeks guidance to organize the learning materials and uses suitable materials
   e. Flexes teaching plan according to the situation.

III. **Implementation**

1. **Implements nursing care competently, safely and accurately within a given time**
   a. Makes appropriate attempts in solving the problems
   b. Carries out nursing intervention appropriately according to priority

c. Encourages patients to utilize own capacities
d. Possesses manual dexterity
e. Works quietly without apparent strain
f. Has self confidence
g. Follows the technique of procedures correctly
h. Demonstrates skill in carrying out basic procedures.

2. **Maintains comfortable environment for patient**
   a. Reduces environment distractions such as bright light, loud noise and staff conversations
   b. Places the patient with a compatible room mate/next bed mate
   c. Provides a comfortable bed ,bed linen is smooth,clean,dry and provides warmth
   d. Personal hygiene needs are met
   e. Shows a concerned and caring attitude
   f. Provides privacy.
3. **Applies scientific principles**
   a. Recalls the underlying scientific principles
   b. Explains the therapeutic effect
   c. Takes precautions wherever necessary
   d. Makes adaptation while following scientific principles
   e. Integrates the scientific principles in giving patient care.
4. **Maintains safe environment**
   a. Provides the unit that is safe, e.g. bed in low position
   b. Places the call bell within easy reach
   c. Instructs the patient how to obtain assistance
   d. Ensures safety while caring for patient, e.g. shifting or ambulating
   e. Observes precautions to provide safety.
5. **Records and reports patients information accurately**
   a. Gives complete reports
   b. Uses appropriate language
   c. Report continuity of care
   d. Decides on specific information to be communicated
   e. Knows to whom the information is to be communicated
   f. Determines the change in patient condition
   g. Records what he/she observes
   h. Follows hospital policy regarding records such as signature, date, time and ink.
6. **Gives health instructions to patients and family**
   a. Reinforce the promotive and preventive aspects of care
   b. Provides and inform about appropriate equipment and resources
   c. Encourages active involvement of patient and family
   d. Considers the factors such as education, age, sex needs and suitable time for the appropriate health teaching.

IV. **Evaluation**

1. **Identifies outcome criteria used to evaluate the patients response to nursing Care**
   a. Identifies data related to outcome criteria
   b. Identifies the response of patients to nursing interventions
   c. Recognizes the specific and observable outcome criteria.
2. **Collects data related to identified criteria**
   a. Data is collected related to physical need
   b. Determines the utilizations of resources
   c. Data related to health teaching given is collected.
3. **Re-examines the patients care plan**
   a. Evaluate the care plan in the light of care given
   b. Observe whether the health teaching plan is implemented
   c. Determines whether the problem has been solved
   d. Determines whether the goals have been achieved.
4. **Modifies the care plan**
   a. Modifies the plan for nursing action based on patient progress
   b. Modifies procedures according to patients response
   c. Communicates the modified plan to the team members verbally
   d. Documents the modified plan
   e. Recognizes the facilities available to improve the planning.

V. **Sense of Responsibility**

1. **Readily accepts responsibility for own behavior, respects rules and regulations**
   a. Assumes responsibility and does the work
   b. Does not need more supervision than the she/he should at his/her level
   c. Is honest, consistent, accountable.

VI. **Initiative for Self-learning**

1. **Eager to learn and seeks new learning experiences**
   a. Eager to learn and seeks new learning experiences
   b. Reports illness on time and keeps fit and alert
   c. Strives for quality improvement
   d. Creative, innovative and imaginative
   e. Able to handle situations intellectually
   f. Initiates positive development
   g. Demonstrates leadership abilities.

VII. **Interpersonal Skills**

1. **Establishes and maintains outstanding working relationships**
   a. Courteous and considerate towards others
   b. Recognizes individual differences
   c. Accepts the differences and uniqeness of each individual

d. Cooperative in assertive manner with co-workers, doctors and other health care team
e. Identifies and accepts the beliefs and practice of others including patients family and community
f. Receptive to suggestions and critisms and attempt to improve
g. Listens to patients, co-workers and seniors
h. Seeks help in difficult situations
i. Expresses herself/himself clearly (verbal and nonverbal).

VIII. **Professional Conduct**

A. **Uniform**

1. **Always well groomed and neat, conscious about professional appearance**
    a. Wears clean uniform according to the uniform regulations
    b. Keeps nails and hands clean
    c. Appears professional in activities and attitudes.

B. **Punctuality**

2. **Exceptionally punctual for clinical and has never been late, completes all given learning assignments on time**
    a. Exceptionally punctual for clinical and has never been late
    b. Completes all given learning assignments on time
    c. Reports any problems related to patient care on time.

The Clinical Effectiveness

What is Clinical Effectiveness and Why it is Important?

Clinical effectiveness is about doing the right things in the right way and at the right time for the right patient. There are several key activities needed to support clinically effective practice

- Selecting a particular aspect of practice to question or examine
- Finding out from the literature and critically apprising this information
- Implementing and/or learning to provide best in clinical practice
- Confirming that providing best practice on day-to-day basis
- Changing practice to make improvements if necessary.

Achieving Clinical Effectiveness

Overall, the three functions involved in achieving clinical effectiveness are ensuring that people know what clinically effective practice is . Applying knowledge about clinically effective practice in day to day patient care and making sure that changes in practice are working to benefit patient.

Clinical Effectiveness MUDEL
Inform
Ensure that nurse patients and managers know the best available evidence of clinical and cost effectiveness
Monitor: Confirm that changes take place locally and result in real improvements in the quality of health care.
Change: Use the information on clinical and cost effectiveness to review, and where necessary, change routine clinical and managerial practice.

Critical Thinking

Think of one area of practice you carry out regularly for patients and consider the following critical thinking:

- Are you certain that you are practicing in a way which is clinically effective for patients that is, the right way to achieve the right result
- Do you know if any research studies have been done to examine different ways of practicing and determine which is best if the research is valid?
- Are there any clinical guidelines available which describe good practice based on research findings and/or expert opinion
- Have you and your colleague discussed and agreed on good practice
- Have you shared your experiences in implementing good practice with colleagues?

Improving Clinical Practice

In recent years, many research studies have confirmed that patients with apparently the same clinical condition are not being treated in the same way across the practioner or places. There is no doubt that this variation in clinical practice exists. Most of this published studies concern medical care. However, it is probable that researchers would find the same levels of variation among the nursing specialties, therapists or any other group of health professionals.

Clinical effectiveness for nurses

Function	Key activities
Inform nurse manager and patient about the available evidence on clinical	Searching the literature and other sources for what makes up good practice • Critically appraising the literature • Seeing if staff are providing what is determined to be good practice on day to day basis • Supporting or carrying out research studies
Change practice where appropriate	Leading or helping to design and implement changes in practice which will result in more clinically effective care.
Monitor practice for change and real improvements in quality and clinical effectiveness	Designing and carrying out clinical audits to see if staffs are providing what is determined to be good practice on a day to day basis

- Do you think that you and all your colleagues carry out the area of practice in the same way for the same patient or do you think there might be some variation in the way you and your colleagues practice
- Could you justify any variation based on sound evidence of what is good practice
- Could you reasonably explain the variation or the resulting variation in the cost of care to members of the public?
- Could you and your colleagues work together to understand your current practice patterns and try to improve them
- Can you and your colleagues check out the sources available to support nurses in improving their practice.

CHAPTER

2

Nursing Assessment for Fundamentals of Nursing

History Taking and General Physical Examination

Name of the student ----------------------------------Course ----------------------

Date ---------------------------------- Clinical posting (Specialty) ----------------

General Patient Information

Name	IP No.
Age	Gender
Marital status	Nationality
Language spoken	Religion
Occupation	Home town/city
Education	Income
Date of admission	Treatment received on arrival to hospital
Provisional diagnosis	Significant lab value

History of Present Illness

Ask any or all of the following as appropriate and write summary below

What problem made you to come to hospital	
When this symptoms started	
Any precipitating factors/aggravating (what were you doing at that time)	
Was the onset sudden or gradual	
How often does the problem occur	
Where is the exact location of the problem	
Has the problem occurred before	
Did you try home or other remedies to cure the problem	
Significant area affected	
Reason for admission	
Direct admission	
Referred by others	

Any relevant information --

Relevant Family History

Type of family: Nuclear/Joint family
Members of the family: Parents/brothers/sisters

Any major illness in the family: Yes/No. If yes specify------------------------------

Who is suffering ---

What disease ---

What is their condition now ---

Past health history
Previous hospitalization
Surgery if any :
History of communicable disease :
Is the client taking any prescription or over the counter medications on a regular basis/ notice all the medications, how long :

Family history of illness
Is there any family history of: Asthma/cancer/diabetes/epilepsy/hypertension/heart disease/ hepatitis/hemophilia/stroke/tuberculosis/mental disorders/aged grand parent and siblings alive? If so what is there current state of health if not state the cause of death and age of death.

Psychosocial and spiritual data
Social support system : Client occupational history. How does illness effect work/study and financial status of the client.

Emotional responses
How does the client appear—happy/sad/anxious/irritable
Body language congruent with what the client saying
Is the client dressed appropriately/clean/unkempt
How does the client feel?
What does the client normally do to cope with disease condition?

Cognitive responses
Does the client have on adequate knowledge of his/her illness and treatment?

Health behaviors
Use of alcohol/tobacco. Does the client comply with therapy/drug abuse.
Does the client comply with therapy?

Values and beliefs
What are the clients attitudes/beliefs about hospitalization?
Does he/she have any in appropriate perception of illness?

General Physical Examination

Use questioning, observation and examination to gather data. Tick items that apply to the client and comment as needed.

Sensation

Eyes

- Poor vision
- Blurred vision
- Eye infection
- Blindness R/L
- Eye pain
- Itching
- Prosthesis
- Glasses/contact lens

Ears

- Ringing in ears
- Discharge
- Ear infection
- Loss of hearing R/L
- Ear pain
- Itching hearing aids

Tongue

Difficulty of taste
- Glossitis
- Stomatitis

Nose

- Frequent colds
- Nose bleeds
- Pain
- Discharge

Touch

Reduced sensation or tactile perception

Comments

Skin and Mucous Membranes

Skin

- Excessive dryness
- Bruising
- Jaundice itching
- Rash
- Broken skin/wound
- Pale/flushed
- Poor turgor
- Change in pigmentation

Mouth and Throat

- Sore throat
- Coated tongue
- Dental caries
- Bad breath (halitosis)
- Bleeding gums
- Dentures upper/lower

Hair

- Itchy scalp
- Hygiene poor
- Dandruff
- Hair change
- Loss/excess

Nails

- Colors changes
- Biting
- Spliting
- Clubbing

Comments

Respiration

Rate ----------------

Characteristics ---------------------------------------

- Cough
- Dyspnea
- Wheezing
- Coughs blood (hemoptysis)
- Cyanosis
- Pain on breathing
- Restlessness
- Smoke (how many per day).

Comments

Circulation

Pulse rate -------------------min Characteristics --

Blood pressure -----------mm Hg

- Fatigue
- Chest pain
- Nausea
- Vomiting
- Anemia
- Varicose veins
- Peripheral pulses
- Leg swelling/ulcers

Comments

Nutrition

Weight -------------------------- Height ---------------------Skin fold thickness -------

- Appetite change
- Weight change
- Nausea vomiting
- Dysphasia
- Heart burn
- Dentures upper/lower

Normal eating pattern (likes and dislikes)

Comments

Abdomen

- Inspection: Rasheses - Lesions - Scar/ striae
- Distended
- Peristalsis - Present/absent - Tenderness/ mass

Elimination

Urinary

- Frequency - Urgency - Dribbling
- Urinary incontinence
- Painful urination - Retention - Dysuria
- Urinary appliance
- Nocturia - Hematuria - Anuria
- Distended bladder

Activity/Exercise

- Muscle pain - Muscle weakness - Cramps
- Joint pain/swelling
- Stiffness of movements - Deformities
- Abnormal gait - Fatigue - Impaired coordination

Self care (describe limitation to eating, bathing, dressing, toileting, ambulating)

Comments

Comfort

Describes the following

Pain if yes how it is relived ---

Sleep pattern and methods/treatment used for sleep ----------------------------

Neurological Responses

- Disorientation - Unconscious - Headache
- Tremors
- Paralysis - Numbness - Weakness
- Seizures (fits)
- Dizziness - Loss of memory
- Difficult expressing self verbally

Comments

Immune Response

Temperature --------------------------------

- Allergies - Fever in last 45 hours - Swollen glands

Chemotherapy---

Sexuality

Female

Age of menarche ------------Last menstrual period (LMP) -----------Duration ------

Flow --------------------Cycle -------------------------- (days)

- Dysmenorrhea - Bleeding between periods
- Vaginal bleeding

Males

- Discharge - Swelling/masses

Comments --

Clinical Evaluation

(Form A)

Name of the student---

Students number ------------------------- Ward------------------------Unit ---------

Group --

Nursing Process

1. Assessment and Diagnosis

Activities	Excellent 4	Very good 3	Good 2	Satisfactory 1	Not satis-factory 0	Not satis-factory	
Collects data about patients needs						Unable to collect data about patients needs	Marks
Identifies basic needs of patients						Unable to identify patients needs	
Categorizes the patients needs/ problems						Unabe to categorize the patients needs	
Formulates nursing diagnosis						Unable to categorize nursing diagnosis	

2. Planning

Activities	Excellent 4	Very good 3	Good 2	Satisfactory 1	Not satis-factory 0	Not satis-factory	
Prioritizes the patient needs						Unable to identify the priority needs	Marks
State the outcome criteria						Unable to state the outcome criteria	

Contd...

Contd...

Activities	Excellent 4	Very good 3	Good 2	Satisfactory 1	Not satisfactory 0	Not satisfactory	
Plans nursing actions for each needs of the patient						Unabe to plan nursing actions for patient or unable to cope with routine work	
States rationale for nursing actions						Unable to state rationale for nursing actions	
Formulates the needed patient health instructions						Makes no attempt to find out the health learning needs of the patients and family	

3. Implementation

Activities	Excellent 4	Very good 3	Good 2	Satisfactory 1	Not satisfactory 0	Not satisfactory	
Implements nursing care competently, safely, and accurately within a given time						In competent to implement nursing care safely and accurately	Marks
Maintains comfortable environment for patient						Ignores body alignment. Does not pay attention to patients discomfort	

Contd...

Contd...

Activities	Excellent 4	Very good 3	Good 2	Satisfactory 1	Not satis-factory 0	Not satis-factory	
Applies scientific principles						Ignores scientific principles when carrying out care	
Maintains safe environment						Unable to maintain healthy, safe and clean environment	
Records and reports patients information accurately						Fails to report or record accurate information	
Gives health instructions to patient and family						Unable to give even incidental teaching to patient and family	

4. Evaluation

Activities	Excellent 4	Very good 3	Good 2	Satisfactory 1	Not satis-factory 0	Not satis-factory	
Identifies outcome criteria used to evaluate the patients response to nursing care						Unable to identify outcome criteria or unable to monitor patients progress	Marks
Collects data related to identified criteria						Unable to collect data related to identified criteria	

Contd...

Contd...

Activities	Excellent 4	Very good 3	Good 2	Satisfactory 1	Not satis-factory 0	Not satis-factory	
Re-examine the patient's care plan						Unable to re-examine the patients care plan	
Modifies the care plan						Unable to modify the care plan	

5. Professional Conduct

a. Uniform

Activities	Excellent 4	Very good 3	Good 2	Satisfactory 1	Not satisfactory 0	Not satis-factory	
Always well groomed and neat, conscious about professional appearance						Pays no attention to grooming and untidy	

b. Punctuality

Activities	Excellent 4	Very good 3	Good 2	Satisfactory 1	Not satis-factory 0	Not satisfactory	
Exceptionally punctual for clinical and has never been late, completes all given learning assignments on time						Consistently late for clinical. Makes no attempt to complete the learning assignments on time. Stops in mid task when clinical hours over	

c. Sense of Responsibility

Activities	Excellent 4	Very good 3	Good 2	Satisfactory 1	Not satis-factory 0	Not satisfactory	
Readily accepts responsibility for own behaviors						Reluctant to take responsibility and avoids it. Breaks rules and regulations	
Respects rules and regulations						Reluctant to take responsibility and avoids it. Breaks rules and regulations	

d. Initiative for Self-learning

Activities	Excellent 4	Very good 3	Good 2	Satisfactory 1	Not satis-factory 0	Not satisfactory	
Eager to learn and seeks new learning experience						Fails to participate in new learning experiences	

e. Interpersonal Skills

Activities	Excellent 4	Very good 3	Good 2	Satisfactory 1	Not satis-factory 0	Not satisfactory	
Establishes and maintains outstanding working relationships						Fails to establish effective working relationship with patients and families	

Total marks: 100. ------- **Marks obtained** -------

Signature of Student ------- **Signature of Clinical Instructor** -------

- Excellent - 4
- Very good - 3
- Good - 2
- Satisfactory - 1
- Not satisfactory - 1

Student Clinical Evaluation

General (Form B)

Name of the student---Year------------------------

Name of the health agency --

Clinical experience from-------------------to---

Sl. No.	Performance criteria	Performance level				
		4	3	2	1	Remarks
	A. Nursing knowledge assessment					
1.	Collect through knowledge about patient's illness					
2.	Recognizes physical needs of the patient					
3.	Categorizes the patient's problem					
4.	Formulate complete nursing diagnosis					
	B. Planning					
5.	Prioritize the patient needs					
6.	Able to organize nursing action within the given time					
	C. Implementation					
7.	Competent in implementing nursing care through safe and accurate, collect and replace the equipment organizing the activities within time					
8.	Maintains comfortable environment for patient					
9.	Accurately records and reports patient information					
	D. Evaluation					
10.	Establishes outcome criteria for the patient including physical state, behaviors and response to treatment					
11.	Able to state rationale for nursing actions					

Contd...

Contd...

Sl. No.	Performance criteria	Performance level				
		4	3	2	1	Remarks
	E. Drug information (knowledge)					
12.	Able to give a description of each drug administered as follow. Name of the drug,action,indications,dosage ranges contraindications, side effects precautions, nurses, responsibilities, etc.					
	F. Diagnosis knowledge					
13.	States accurate medical diagnosis of each patient cared for and describes etiology, signs and symptoms, medical therapy result of medical therapy					
	G. Laboratory investigations					
14.	States proper name of laboratory investigations of each patient. Each patient cared for and describes reasons for tests, patient preparation for test, test procedure					
	H. Teaching skill					
15.	Identifies health teaching needs of patient					
16.	Involve patient and family in all phases of teaching					
	I. Leadership and management skill					
17.	Is knowledgeable about the organizations structure					
18.	Manages recourses in a cost effective manner					
	J. Professional conduct					
19.	Uniform: Always well groomed and neat, conscious about professional appearance					

Contd...

Contd...

Sl. No.	Performance criteria	Performance level				
		4	3	2	1	Remarks
	K. Punctuality					
20.	Exceptionally punctual for clinical and has never been late, completes all given learning assignments in time					
21.	Readily accepts responsibilities, reliable, adaptable and displays consistency in work,judgement in consistently sound and logical					
	L. Communication skills					
22.	Patient and family: Establishes and maintenance outstanding working with relationship with patients and families					
23.	Hospital staff/Health team: Establishes harmonious relationship with the member of health team					
24.	Initiative for self learning: Eager to learn and seek new learning experiences					
25.	Teacher: Always respect teachers and accepts constructive criticisms					

Total marks: 100. ---------------- **Total marks obtained ----------------**

Signature of Student----------------------------

Signature of Clinical Instructor-------------------

Key:

- Very good-4
- Good-3
- Satisfactory-2
- Not satisfactory-1

Unit Orientation Accident and Emergency Services

Sl. No.	Skills	Performance satisfactory	Performance unsatisfactory	Preceptors/ clinical instructor initial	Date	Comments of mentor
1.	Registration of patient in accident and emergency a. Registration desk b. First registration c. Patient seen before d. Critically ill patient e. Referred patient					
2.	Admission a. Obtained bed b. Physician informed c. Record maintained					
3.	Valuables belongings a. Policies and procedures b. Admitted patient c. Accompanied patient d. Unaccompanied patient					
4.	Ability to keep allocated work area stocked with necessary equipment and ready for use a. Emergency equipment b. Oxygen c. Monitors d. Defibrillator e. Suction f. Intubation set g. IV set ready h. Crash cart i. Room checklist					
5.	Follow policy and procedures regarding patients brought in dead					

Contd...

Contd...

Sl. No.	Skills	Performance satisfactory	Performance unsatisfactory	Preceptors/ clinical instructor initial	Date	Comments of mentor
6.	Physical assessment of patients a. Vital signs b. Neurological status					
7.	Triage The triage nurse is responsible for informing the charge nurse/nursing supervisor of all patients brought into the department from the ambulatory care area for further care. A brief report should be given outlining the patient sex ,age, chief complaint and general condition. The charge nurse / nursing supervisor are responsible for keeping the triage nurse informed of bed available in the department. a. Set nursing priorities and allocate rooms appropriately b. Triage of accident and emergency patient c. All patient presenting should be assessed if their condition requires immediate or non-urgent Intervention. This is the primary responsibility of the triage nurse d. Prioritizing care					

Contd...

Contd...

Sl. No.	Skills	Performance satisfactory	Performance unsatisfactory	Preceptors/ clinical instructor initial	Date	Comments of mentor
	e. The triage nurse is further responsible for ensuring that the urgent needs of patient are met promptly after prioritizing patients needs. She/he should communicate those needs to charge nurse or physician as appropriate f. Allocation of rooms the triage nurse is responsible for assigning the care area appropriate to the patient's needs					
8.	Cardiopulmonary resusititation –CODE accident and emergency nurse should be currently certified and able to perform effective BCLS/CPR					
9.	Cardiac monitoring: accident and emergency nurse should be able to recognize all life threatening arrhythmia's					
10.	Set up and use suction equipment					
11.	Set up and administer oxygen therapy a. General considerations b. Assessment of patient c. Monitoring oxygen therapy					

Contd...

Contd...

Sl. No.	Skills	Performance satisfactory	Performance unsatisfactory	Preceptors/ clinical instructor initial	Date	Comments of mentor
12.	Initiate and maintain IV infusion a. Calculation b. Intake and output chart c. Documentation					
13.	Initiate and maintain blood transfusion					
14.	Administration of medication as per protocol					
15.	Obtain specimens a. Urine specimen b. Blood specimen c. Wound specimen.C&S d. Stool specimen e. Throat specimen. C&S					
16.	Demonstrate correct lifting techniques. a. Ambulatory b. Non ambulatory c. Spinal injury					
17.	First aid skills: a. support dressing b. bandages c. slings cervical collars					
18.	Perform urinary catheterization					
19.	Perform NGT insertion					
20.	Prepare patient for operation a. special consideration in accident and emergency					

Total marks: 100. ------- **Total marks obtained** -------

Signature of Student ------- **Signature of Clinical Instructor** -------

- Very good - 4
- Good - 3
- Satisfactory - 2
- Not satisfactory - 1

Medication Proficiency

Sl. No.	Skills	Performance unsatisfactory	Performance satisfactory	Date	Preceptor's initials	Comments
1.	Administration of medication					
2.	Controlled drugs follow policy, procedures					
3.	Maintain narcotic box					
4.	Filling out prescription					
5.	Obtaining narcotics					
6.	Administer piggy-back intravenous medications					
7.	Insertion into a vein for intravenous therapy					
8.	Administration of routine intravenous solutions and dressing change					
9.	Administering medication following proper procedure • Oral • Eye drops/ ointment • Ear drops/ instillation • Nasal drops • Rectal suppository • Subcutaneous /intradermal • Intramuscular • Intravenous					

Contd...

Contd...

Sl. No.	Skills	Performance unsatisfactory	Performance satisfactory	Date	Preceptor's initials	Comments
10.	Medication calculation adult single dose					
11.	Intravenous calculation • Infusion rate • Infused volume					
12.	Drawing up insulin • Regular insulin • NPH insulin • Recording insulin site location chart • Unit calculation • Recording regular ordered medication					

Signature of Student----------------------------

Signature of Clinical Instructor-------------------

Clinical Assessment Tool: Vital Signs

Recording Vital Signs

Sl. No.	Activities	1= Satisfactory	0=Unsatisfactory	Not assessed
1.	**Assessment**			
	Determine need to measure vital signs			
2.	Assess for signs and symptoms of vital signs alteration			
3.	Assess for factors that normally influence vital signs			
4.	Assess factors affecting the timing of temperature and pulse taking			
5.	Identify patients baseline of vital signs from the record			
6.	Determine appropriate sites for measurement of temperature, pulse and blood pressure			
	Implementation			
7.	Collected all equipment for vital signs measurement			
8.	Explained assessment procedure to the patient			
9.	Placed the patient in an appropriate position (sitting or supine)			
10.	Provided for patients privacy			
11.	Washed hands before starting the procedures			
	Temperature, pulse, respiration			
12.	Read mercury level while gently rotating thermometer at eye level			
13.	Shook thermometer down briskly to proper level (below 35.5°C).			

Contd...

Contd...

Sl. No.	Activities	1= Satisfactory	0=Unsatisfactory	Not assessed
14.	Asked the patient to open mouth and gently placed thermometer under tongue (oral)			
15.	Moved clothing or gown away from patients shoulder and arm (axilla)			
16.	Inserted thermometer correctly (axilla)			
17.	Positioned the arm for taking pulse			
18.	Placed finger tips of first three fingers over radial pulse			
19.	Palpated patients radial pulse			
20.	Counted pulse rate for complete 1 minute			
21.	Assessed regularity and frequency of any dysrhythmia			
22.	Determined strength and character of pulse			
23.	Positioned patient and self properly to ensure view of chest wall movement			
24.	Observed complete respiratory cycle			
25.	Correctly counted respiration for complete 1 minute			
26.	Assessed respiratory depth			
27.	Assessed respiratory rhythm			
28.	Removed thermometer after 2 minutes or according to the hospital policy (oral)			
29.	Wiped off secretions from stem to bulb with tissue. Discarded			
30.	Read while gentle rotating thermometer at eye level			

Contd...

Contd...

Sl. No.	Activities	1= Satisfactory	0=Unsatisfactory	Not assessed
31.	Washed thermometer in lukewarm soapy water, rinsed, dried, and replaced in storage container			
	Blood pressure			
32.	Positioned patients forearm at heart level with palm of hand turned up			
33.	Removed constricting clothing from around upper arm			
34.	Palpated brachial artery			
35.	Positioned cuff properly above brachial artery, and wrapped deflated cuff evenly and snuggly around the upper arm			
36.	Positioned manometer correctly for viewing			
37.	Identified approximate systolic pressure by palpating brachial or radial pulse during cuff inflation			
38.	Checked stethoscope amplification of sounds			
39.	Applied stethoscope correctly over brachial artery			
40.	Tightened valve of pressure bulb			
41.	Correctly inflated cuff to 30 mm Hg above that of palpated systolic			
42.	Allowed mercury to fall evenly at rate of 2 to 3 mm Hg/sec during auscultation			
43.	Noted point on manometer when first clear sound was heard accurately			
44.	Continued to deflate cuff gradually, noting point at which sound disappeared accurately			

Contd...

Contd...

Sl. No.	Activities	1= Satisfactory	0=Unsatisfactory	Not assessed
45.	Rapidly deflated cuff completely and removed from patients arm			
46.	When blood pressure was inaudible or difficult to obtain, repeated measurement after waiting 1–2 minutes			
47.	Assisted patient in returning to comfortable position			
48.	Recorded vital signs correctly on vital signs flow sheet/ progress sheet			
49.	Replaced all equipment to its normal location			
50.	Washed hands after the procedure			

Total =

General comments

Signature of Student-----------------------------

Signature of Clinical Supervisor--

CHAPTER

3a Nursing Care Plan Format

History Taking and Physical Examination

Nursing assessment frequency and extent of the nursing assessment of any system function are based on several factors, including the severity of the patient's symptoms and presence of risk factors, the purpose of assessment.

The physical examination is used to determine the strengths of the patient or the responses the patient exhibits:

Nursing History

Name of the nursing institute --

Student name --

Specialty posting ----------------------Period from----------------to----------

Demographic Data

Name of the patient	IP No.
Age	Gender
Marital status	Nationality
Language spoken	Religion
Occupation	Home town/city
Education	Income
Date of admission	Treatment received on arrival to hospital
Provisional diagnosis	Name of the Doctor who is treating the patient ------------------------------ And unit ---------------------------

History of Present Illness

Ask any or all of the following as appropriate and write a summary

Date of admission --

Reason for visit --

When did the symptoms started---

General state of health ---

Was the onset sudden or gradual ---

How often the problem occurs --

Has the problem occur before ---

Summary ---

Treatment received on arrival to hospital ---

Chief Complaint

Eliciting a client's history not only assist with individualizing the plan of care but also helps to establish a bond with that client.

Gather specific information regarding onset, location, duration, characteristics, associated manifestation, aggravating and relieving factors.

As a medical surgical nursing nurse standing at the client bed side you may be the first one to see the client and obtain the history.

Onset --

Location --

Duration --

Aggravating factors---

Relieving factors ---

Associated manifestation ---

Past surgical history--

Past medical history --

Allergies --

Medication History

Medication prescribed. Use of anti-hypertensive/diuretics/vasodilator nitroglycerin/anticoagulant/digoxin/bronchodilators/contraceptive/ hormones/steroids/anti-depressant/psychotropic/thyroid hormones/over the counter medication/herbs.
Note time and dosage and how often they are taking.

Allergies

Note and describe any environmental, food or drug allergies.

Relevant Family History

Type of family: Nuclear/joint family

Members of the family: Parents/brothers/sisters ---------------------------------

Family history of illness
Is there any family history of: Asthma/cancer/diabetes/epilepsy/hypertension/heart disease/ hepatitis/hemophilia/stroke/tuberculosis/mental disorders/ thyroid or autoimmune disorders aged grand parent and siblings alive? If so what is there current state of health if not state the cause of death and age of death

Any major illness in the family: Yes/ No. If yes specify------------------------------

Who is suffering --

What disease ---

What is their condition now --

Past health history
Previous hospitalization
Surgery if any :
History of communicable disease :
Is the client taking any prescription or over the counter medications on a regular basis/ notice all the medications, how long :

Psychosocial and spiritual data
Social support system : Client occupational history. How does illness effect work/study and financial status of the client.

Emotional responses
How does the client appear—happy/sad/anxious/irritable
Body language congruent with what the client saying
Is the client dressed appropriately/clean/unclean
How does the client feel
What does the client normally do to cope with disease condition

Cognitive responses
Does the client have on adequate knowledge of his/her illness and treatment

Health behaviors
Use of alcohol/tobacco. Does the client comply with therapy/drug abuse
Does the client comply with therapy

Values and beliefs
What are the clients attitudes/beliefs about hospitalization?
Does he/she have any in appropriate perception of illness?

Dietary Habits

Assess excess or deficit caloric intake and clients approximate intake of foods, high in sodium, cholesterol, saturated fat, and caffeine.

Physical Examination

Use questioning, observation and examination to gather data. Tick items that apply to the client and comment as needed.

Sensation

Eyes

- Poor vision
- Blurred vision
- Eye infection
- Blindness R/L
- Eye Pain
- Itching
- Prosthesis
- Glasses/contact lens

Ears

- Ringing in ears
- Discharge
- Ear infection
- Loss of hearing R/L
- Ear pain
- Itching
- Hearing aids

Tongue

Difficulty of taste

Nose

- Frequent colds
- Nose bleeds
- pain
- Discharge

Touch

Reduced or tactile perception

Comments

Skin and Mucous Membranes

Skin

- Excessive dryness
- Bruising
- Jaundice
- Itching
- Rash
- Broken skin/wound
- Pale/flushed
- Poor turgor
- Change in pigmentation

Mouth and Throat

- Sore throat
- Coated tongue
- Dental caries
- Bad breath (halitosis)
- Bleeding gums
- Dentures upper/lower

Hair

- Itchy scalp
- Hygiene poor
- Dandruff
- Hair change
- Loss/excess

Nails

- Color changes
- Biting
- Spliting
- Clubbing

Comments

Respiration

Rate ----------------

Characteristics --

- Cough
- Dyspnea
- Wheezing
- Coughs blood (hemoptysis)
- Cyanosis
- Pain on breathing
- Restlessness
- Smoke (how many per day)

Comments

Circulation

Pulse rate -------------------/min; Characteristics ------------------------------------

Blood pressure -----------mm Hg

- Fatigue
- Chest pain
- Nausea
- Vomiting
- Anemia
- Varicose veins
- Peripheral pulses
- Leg swelling/ulcers

Comments

Nutrition

Weight -------------------------- Height ---------------------Skin fold thickness -----

- Appetite change
- Weight change
- Nausea
- Vomiting
- Dysphasia
- Heart burn
- Dentures upper/lower

Normal eating pattern (likes and dislikes)

Comments

Abdomen

- Inspection: Rasheses
- Lesions
- Scar/striae
- Distended
- Peristalsis: present/absent
- Tenderness/mass

Elimination

Urinary

- Frequency - Urgency - Dribbling
- Urinary incontinence
- Painful urination - Retentation - Dysuria
- Urinary appliance
- Nocturia - Hematuria - Anuria
- Distended bladder

Activity/Exercise

- Muscle pain - Muscle weakness - Cramps
- Joint pain/swelling
- Stiffness of movements - Deformities
- Abnormal gait - Fatigue - Impaired coordination

Self care (describe limitation to eating, bathing, dressing, toileting, ambulating)

Comments

Comfort

Describes the following

Pain, if yes, how it is relived?

Sleep pattern and methods/treatment used for sleep

Neurological Responses

- Disorientation - Unconscious - Headache
- Tremors
- Paralysis - Numbness - Weakness
- Seizures (fits)
- Dizziness - Loss of memory
- Difficult expressing self verbally

Comments

Immune Response

Temperature --------------------------------

- Allergies
- Fever in last 45 hours
- Swollen glands

Chemotherapy---

Comments

Sexuality

Female

Age of menarche ----------------------LMP ----------------------Duration --------

Flow --------------------Cycle ------------------------- (days)

- Dysmenorrheal
- Bleeding between periods
- Vaginal bleeding

Males

- Discharge
- Swelling/masses

Comments

Investigation Done

Date	Name of the investigation	Normal values	Patients values/result	Significance

Medical diagnosis (final) --

Drug Management

Name of the drug	Dosage and frequency	Route	Action	Side effect	Nursing Intervention

Diet Plan

24 Hours Nutritional Requirements

Type of diet required (snacks, lunch, dinner)

Time	`Type	Quantity	Frequency	Remarks

List of Nursing Diagnosis/Problems/Need Identified according to Priority

1. --
2. --
3. --
4. --
5. --
6. --
7. --
8. -- ----------------------
9. --

Nursing Care Plan

Minimum of 5 problems should be addressed in your care plan

Nursing assessment (observation)	Nursing diagnosis	Objectives	Nursing intervention /action	Rationale	Evaluation
Subjective data What patient complains (symptoms) Objective data What nurse observes (signs)			Carrying planned nursing actions	Scientific principles	Problem resolved /result of intervention

Conclusion

Health education

CHAPTER

3b Nursing Case Study Format

Nursing care study format includes (pls refer page no. 39–46, Unit 3a):

- History taking and physical examination
- Demographic data
- History of present illness
- Chief complaint
- Medication history
- Relevant family history
- Past health history
- Physical examination

Compare Patient Condition with Theory Knowledge of Disease Condition Wherever Applicable

Diagnosis --

	Theory knowledge of disease condition of patient	Present patient condition
Definition		
Related anatomy and physiology		
Etiology		
Risk factors		
Clinical manifestation		

Contd...

Contd...

	Theory knowledge of disease condition of patient	Present patient condition
Pathophysiology		

Investigation Done

Date	Name Investigation	Normal values	Patient values/ result	Significance

Medical Diagnosis:...

Medical Management...

Drug Management

Name of the drug	Dosage and frequency	Route	Action	Side effect	Nursing intervention

Diet Plan

Type of diet required (Snacks, launch, dinner)

Time	Type	Quantity	Frequency	Remarks

List of Nursing Diagnosis/Problems/Need/Identified According to Priority

Nursing Care Plane

Nursing assessment	Nursing diagnosis	Objectives	Nursing interventions	Rationale	Evaluation
Subjective data: When patient complaint symptoms **Objectives data:** What nurse observes (Sign)			Carrying plan nursing actions	Scientific principles	Problem resolved result of intervention

Summary..

Conclusion...

Health education...

Reference..

CHAPTER

4

Performance Evaluation of General Nursing Procedures

Performance Evaluation: Admitting Client to Nursing Unit

Sl. No.	Performance Criteria	S	U	NP	Comments
	Assessment				
1.	Room preparation : Prepared room, equipments, furniture, and bed				
2.	Assessed any special equipment such as suction or oxygen supplies are required				
3.	Greeted client and family cordially introduced self by name and job title				
	Implementation				
1.	Escorted client and family to assigned room, introduced patient to roommates and new environment				
2.	Explained the use of lockers, bed television, telephone, call light/bell, emergency signals and bathroom.				
3.	Explained policies related to no smoking, visiting hours and meals				
4.	Assessed the client general appearance, noting signs and symptoms of physical distress				
5.	Oriented client to nursing division				
6.	Checked personal property and maintained appropriate records of the valuable				
7.	Explained purpose and schedule of planned treatment and procedure				
8.	Completed admission procedures (bed no, identification band/IP No)				
9.	Completed the nursing assessment form and admission record.				

Contd...

Contd...

Sl. No.	Performance Criteria	S	U	NP	Comments
10.	Checked baseline vital signs and recorded it in appropriate records.				
11.	Checked physician order, progress notes and other documents for prompt treatment				
12.	Informed attending physician of the arrival of the patient.				
13.	Notified catering department on new arrival of the patient for arranging food				
14.	Activated appropriate nursing care plan				
	Evaluation				
1.	Observed the comfort of patient				
2.	Monitored patient ability to ambulate independently				
	Recording				
1.	Recorded time of admission and unit in admission register				
2.	Informed nurse in-charge about patient arrival				

Signature of student ---------------------------------------

Signature of clinical instructor --------------------------------

Performance Evaluation: Transferring Client to a Different Nursing Unit/Agency

Sl. No.	Performance Criteria	S	U	NP	Comments
	Assessment				
1.	Determined reason for transfer alone or in collaboration with patient physician(e.g. change in patient condition, availability of speciality,resource available at agency, patient/ family preferences regarding patient location)				
2.	Assessed patients current physical condition and determine vehicle for transport				
3.	Assessed/ determined method for transport. (e.g. wheel chair or stretcher)				
	Planning				
1.	Maintaining patient physical well-being during transport to nursing unit				

Contd...

Contd...

Sl. No.	Performance Criteria	S	U	NP	Comments
2.	Safe transport and care of patient personal belongings				
3.	Obtaining transfer orders from sending physician, including receiving physicians particulars				
4.	Arranging equipment required for transfer				
	Implementation				
1.	Gathered patient personal belongings				
2.	Verified all documentation including care plan is completed and current in- patient medical record				
3.	Collected medical record, medication tickets and other related records				
4.	Performed final assessment to patient physical stability(i.e. check vital signs, check for clear airway, inspect patency of intravenous lines, note patient level of consciousness				
5.	Determined if receiving unit is preferred to accept patient				
6.	Informed patient arrival and introduce patient to nurse assuming care				
7.	Provided verbal report of patient's current condition to nurse in receiving unit, like major therapies being received e.g. oxygen, intravenous fluids, pending treatment or procedures ordered for day and any special nursing care needs.				
8.	Handed over patient record to receiving nurse				
9.	Observed receiving nurse documents clients arrival in nurses notes by recording date and time of arrival, method of transport, patients condition and care provided				
	Follow up activities				
1.	Observed receiving nurse assist client in the new environment/unit				
2.	Observed receiving nurse reviews client record and implement ordered treatments or procedures				

Signature of Student ---------------------------------------

Signature of Clinical Instructor -------------------------------

Performance Evaluation: Discharging Dependent Client from a Health Care Agency

Sl. No.	Performance Criteria	S	U	NP	Comments
	Assessment				
1.	Collaborated with physician and other disciplines in assessing need for referral or discharging to home				
2.	Checked physician discharge orders for prescription, change in treatment etc.				
3.	Determined whether patient or family are ready with transport.				
4.	Identified the need for health teaching related to therapies to administer at home and follow up visits and explained the same				
5.	Assessed patient acceptance of health problems and related restrictions				
	Nursing diagnosis				
1.	Formulated diagnosis based on subjective and objective data • Ineffective therapeutic management related to self care activities • Anxiety related to impending discharge				
	Planning				
1.	Developed individualized goals for patient discharge. Based on nursing diagnosis • Client will be able to care for individualized needs • Patient home environment will be safe				
	Implementation				
1.	Conducted teaching sessions related to health care needs, treatment regimens, and the physical signs or symptoms to be reported to physician				

Contd...

Contd...

Sl. No.	Performance Criteria	S	U	NP	Comments
2.	Offered assistance as patient dresses and packs all personal belongings				
3.	Confirmed with significant others for account settlement				
4.	Obtained wheel chair for patient to shift to transport				
5.	Used proper body mechanics and transfer techniques in assisting patient to wheel chair				
6.	Escorted patient to entrance of institute where source of transport was waiting				
	Recording and reporting				
1.	Completed documentation of status of client health problems at the time of discharge				
2.	Documented client discharge				
3.	Notified house keeping of need to clean client room				

Signature of Student ---------------------------------------

Signature of Clinical Instructor ------------------------------

Performance Evaluation: Making Unoccupied Bed

	Performance Criteria	S	U	NP	Comments
	Assessment				
1.	Assessed need for bed making				
2.	Assembled and arranged equipment at bed side table				
	Implementation				
1.	Washed hands				
2.	Put on the disposable gloves				
3.	Adjusted the bed height to a comfortable working position and lowered the side rail				
4.	Loosen all linen from head to toe				

Contd...

Contd...

	Performance Criteria	S	U	NP	Comments
5.	Folded and kept revisable linen such as blanket, bed spread on bed side table				
6.	Bundled all soiled linen and directly placed in to the laundry bag				
7.	Brought mattress towards the head of the bed				
8.	Placed bottom sheet with its center fold in center of bed and towards the top				
9.	Unfolded the bottom sheet, spread it over the mattress and tucked in with mitered corner				
10.	Placed the draw sheet and tuck it along side				
11.	Moved to the opposite side and tucked the sheets in the same manner				
12.	Returned to the side of the bed first made and placed the top sheet with its centered fold in the center of the bed. Unfolded it with the top edge even with the top of the mattress and spread excess sheet over the bottom edge of the mattress				
13.	Placed the blanket over the top sheet about 6 inches below the top of the sheet				
14.	Tucked the top sheet, blanket and bed spread under the foot of the bed on the side close and miter the corners				
15.	Folded the upper 6 inches of the top sheet down over the spread and made a cuff				
16.	Moved to the other side of the bed and followed the same procedure for screening top sheets				
17.	Kept the pillow case and placed the pillow at the end with the open end away from the entrance				
18.	Fan folded the top linens				
19.	Rearranged the furniture's and placed personal items within easy reach				
20.	Adjusted the bed to a comfortable height for the client				
21.	Disposed off soiled linen and washed hands				

Contd...

Contd...

	Performance Criteria	S	U	NP	Comments
	Record and reporting				
1.	Reported bed making to nurse incharge				

Signature of Student ---------------------------------------

Signature of Clinical Instructor -------------------------------

Performance Evaluation: Making Occupied Bed

	Performance Criteria	S	U	NP	Comments
	Assessment				
1.	Explained the procedure to client and identified the client physical ability				
2.	Washed hands and put on gloves				
3.	Assembled equipment and arranged on the bedside chair in proper order and removed unnecessary equipment				
4.	Closed door and drawn bedside curtain				
5.	Adjusted the bed heights to a comfortable working position				
6.	Lowered the side rail on one side of bed				
7.	Loosened all top linen and removed bedspread and blanket separately				
8.	Folded and placed on the bed side table				
9.	Shifted mattress up to the head of bed				
10.	Assisted the client to turn toward the opposite side and repositioned the pillow under the client head				
11.	Loosen all bottom linens and fan folded soiled linens as far from the client as possible				
12.	Placed the clean bottom sheet length wise making sure that that middle fold is in the middle of the bed and vertically fanfold the half toward the center of the bed				
13.	Tucked the head end, mitered corners and tucked sides				

Contd...

Contd...

	Performance Criteria	S	U	NP	Comments
14.	Placed the clean draw sheet on the center of the bed, fan folded upper half vertically toward the center of the bed. Tucked the side edge under the mattress.				
15.	Raised side rail on working side and moved to the other side				
16.	Lowered side rail. Assisted the client to roll slowly onto the other side over folds of linen, repositioned the pillow and top sheet				
17.	Loosened and removed all bottom linen and placed them in a linen bag				
18.	Spreaded cleanly, fan folded linen smoothly over the edge of the mattress and tucked it from head to foot				
19.	Assisted the client to turn on the back and repositioned the pillow				
20.	Placed a clean top sheet over the client with centerfold lengthwise down middle of bed. Unfolded over client and asked the client to hold clean top sheet or tuck the sheet around the client shoulders. Removed the soiled top sheet and collected it in a linen bag				
21.	Placed blanket over the top sheet and unfolded to cover the client by making sure that the top sheet is kept 6 to 8 inches extra from the edge of blanket				
22.	Placed and unfold bedspread over blanket extending top edge of spread about 2 inches above blanket edge. Tucked top edge of spread over and under edge of blanket				
23.	Turned the edge of top sheet down over the top edge of blanket and spread				
24.	Tucked the foot end of top linen under mattress giving enough freedom for movement				
25.	Raised side rail lowered the bed height to a comfortable position				
26.	Changed pillow cases and placed them in position. Replaced the comfort devices in place, rearranged furniture and opened bedside curtain				

Contd...

Contd...

	Performance Criteria	S	U	NP	Comments
27.	Disposed the soiled linen according to the hospital policy and washed hands				
	Recording and reporting				
1.	Reported bed making to nurse incharge				

Signature of student ---------------------------------------

Signature of Clinical Instructor --------------------------------

Performance Evaluation: Performing General Survey

The general survey is the preliminary portion of the examination, during which the client vital signs, height and weight, skin fold thickness, and general behavior and appearance are recorded, before detailed physical examination.

Sl. No.	Performance Criteria	S	U	NP	Comments
	Assessment				
1.	Assessed client general perception about personal health				
2.	Discussed client health history such as • History of illness • Reasons for visiting hospital • Recent weight gain/loss • Alteration in vital signs • Diet habit • Type of diet • Type of exercise • Fluid intake • Checked dress proper for physical exam • Observed appearance and verbal expression and posture				
	Nursing diagnosis				
1.	Anxiety related to hospitalization Observed related factors based on assessment data				
	Planning				
1.	Developed individualized goals based on nursing diagnosis				
	Implementation				
1.	Explained procedure to client				

Contd...

Contd...

Sl. No.	Performance Criteria	S	U	NP	Comments
2.	Measured/ recorded vital signs, height and weight of the client				
3.	Assessed skin fold thickness				
4.	Observed and recorded hygiene and grooming				
5.	Performed specific nursing assessment based on client health problem/needs				
	Evaluation				
1.	Compared client, vital signs, height, weight and emotional behavior with normal range				
2.	Compared client skin fold thickness with 50th percentile				
	Recording and reporting				
1.	Recorded vital signs on flow sheet				
2.	Recorded client height and weight in nurses notes				
3.	Recorded description and skin fold thickness				
4.	Reported abnormalities to physician				
5.	Reported abnormalities to in charge nurse				

Signature of Student ---------------------------------------

Signature of Clinical Instructor ------------------------------

Performance Evaluation: Maintaining Body Alignment

Body alignment refers to the conditions of the joints, tendons ligaments and muscle in various body positions. When the body is aligned, when standing, sitting, or lying no excessive strain is put to these structures. Body alignment contributes to body balance. Without this balance, the center gravity is displaced, which increases the force of gravity. The person is consequently at risk for falling and receiving an injury.

Sl. No.	Performance Criteria	S	U	NP	Comments
	Assessment				
1.	Observed alignment of client in standing, sitting and lying position as **Standing** • Head is erect and at midline • Shoulders and hips are straight and parallel • Vertebral column appears straight **Lateral observation** • Documents that abdomen is comfortable, tucked in and knees and ankles are flexed • Arms are comfortably positioned at each side • Feet are placed slightly apart, with toes pointed forward • Center of gravity is located midline				
	Sitting • Head is erect ,and vertebrae are in straight alignment • Body weight is evenly distributed on buttocks and thighs **Lying** • Client is in lateral position, with positioning supports removed • Client's body is supported by adequate mattress • Vertebral column is in alignment without observable curves				
	Nursing diagnosis				
1.	Impaired physical mobility				
	Planning				
1.	Client will assume positions that maintain musculoskeletal alignment				
	Client will understand how and why to assume body alignment				
	Implementation				
1.	Instructed client and family on proper alignment for standing, sitting or lying				
2.	Demonstrated to client and family correct body alignment for standing, sitting and lying				
3.	Discussed with client and family hazards of prolonged immobility on body alignment and mobility				

Contd...

Contd...

Sl. No.	Performance Criteria	S	U	NP	Comments
	Evaluation				
1.	Inspected skin surfaces				
2.	Encouraged client to describe the benefit of body alignment				
	Recording and reporting				
1.	Recorded information presented to client and progresses				
2.	Reported to charge nurse information taught to client				

Signature of Student ---------------------------------------

Signature of Clinical Instructor ------------------------------

Performance Evaluation: Using Safe and Effective Transfer Technique

Transferring is a nursing skill that helps the dependent client attains positions to regain optimum independence as quickly as possible. Physical activity maintains and improves joint motion, increase strength, promotes circulation, relieves pressure on skin, and improves urinary and respiratory functions. It also benefits the client psychologically by increasing social activity and mental stimulation and providing a change in environment. Thus, mobilization plays a crucial role in the client rehabilitation.

One of the major concerns during transfer is the safety of the client and nurse. The nurse prevents self injury by using good posture, minimal muscle strength, and effective body mechanics and lifting techniques.

The nurse must be aware of the client motor deficits, ability to aid in transfer, and body weight as rule of thumb. Nurses should never attempt to lift more than 35% of their body weight and must always get assistance if in doubt about their ability to transfer a client.

Sl. No.	Performance Criteria	S	U	NP	Comments
	Assessment				
1.	Assessed physiologic capacity to transfer such as • Muscle strength(legs and upper arms) • Joint mobility and contracture formation • Paralysis or paresis (spastic or flaccid) • Bone continuity(trauma, amputation)				

Contd...

Contd...

Sl. No.	Performance Criteria	S	U	NP	Comments
2.	Assessed level of endurance, such as • Ability to use arms and legs for moving • Posture and changes in equilibrium • Ability to maintain balance while sitting in bed or on side of bed • Client sensory status, adequacy of vision, adequacy of earing • Pain • Ability to follow verbal instruction • Client specific risk of falling when transferring.				
	Nursing diagnosis				
1.	• Impaired physical mobility • High risk for injury				
	Planning				
1.	Client will not suffer injury or discomfort during transfer				
2.	Client will demonstrate increased activity tolerance				
	Implementation				
1.	Washed hands				
2.	Assisted client in sitting position				
3.	Placed client in supine position				
4.	Removed pillows				
5.	Placed feet apart with foot nearer bed behind other foot				
6.	Placed hand farther from client under shoulders, supporting client's head and cervical vertebrae				
7.	Placed other hand on bed surface, raised client to sitting position by shifting weight from front to black leg				
8.	Assisted client to sitting position on side of bed • Stood opposite to client hips, and turned diagonally • Placed arm nearer head of bed under client shoulders, supporting head and neck • Remained in front until client regain balance • Lowered level of bed until client feet touches the floor				

Contd...

Contd...

Sl. No.	Performance Criteria	S	U	NP	Comments
9.	Transferred client from bed to chair • Assisted client to sitting position on side of bed • Placed chair in position at 45o degree angle to bed • Ensured client stable leg is placed forward with weak foot back • Spread feet apart • Rocked client to standing on count of three while straightening hips and legs, knee slightly flexed. • Assessed client for proper alignment in sitting position				
10.	Transferred from bed to stretcher • Three nurses stood side by side facing side of client bed • Each person assumed responsibility for one of the three areas, head and shoulders, hips and thighs and ankles. • Each assumed wide base of support with foot closer to stretcher in front, knees slightly flexed • Lifters arms are placed under client head and shoulders, hips and thighs and ankles, with fingers securely around other side of client body • Lifters, roll client towards their chests and on count of three, client is shifted and held against nurses chest • On second count of three, nurses step back and pivot toward stretcher, moving forward • Nurses gently lowerd client onto center of stretcher by flexing knees and hips until elbows are level with edge of stretcher				
11.	Nurses assessed client body alignment, placed safety straps across body, and raised side rails				
12.	Positioned chair near bed and allowed adequate space to maneuver lift				
	Evaluation				
1.	Observed for correct body alignment, enquired client experienced any pain during transfer				

Contd...

Contd...

Sl. No.	Performance Criteria	S	U	NP	Comments
	Record and report				
1.	Recorded procedure in nurses notes				
2.	Reported to physician about client transfer				

Signature of Student ---------------------------------------

Signature of Clinical Instructor --------------------------------

Performance Evaluation: Assessment of Thyroid Gland

Sl. No.	Performance Criteria	S	U	NP	Comments
1.	**Assessment** Enquired client has history of recent bodily changes. General or Local				
2.	Assessed, history of thyroid problems or takes thyroid medication				
	Nursing diagnosis				
1.	Nursing diagnosis based on assessment data				
	Planning				
1.	Determined presence of abnormalities, signs of thyroid masses				
	Implementation				
1.	Explained procedure to client Washed hands				
2.	Observed the lower neck region				
3.	Draw curtains/ screen around client				
4.	Inspected the patients neck identifying the thyroid gland cricoids cartilage, trachea and sternocleidomastoid muscles				
5.	Inspected area of lower neck overlying the thyroid gland for symmetry and visible masses				
6.	Anterior approach Asked client to extend neck slightly and swallow. Observe for presence of any bulging				

Contd...

Contd...

Sl. No.	Performance Criteria	S	U	NP	Comments
7.	A glass of water offered to the client. Watch the neck during swallowing. Informed the client to lower his chin slightly				
8.	Standing in front of the client, use the pads of middle and index fingers to locate the cricoid cartilage. Ask him to swallow than feel for the thyroid isthmus. Note for any enlargement nodules or irregularities				
9.	Have the patient flex his head slightly forward and to the right to palpate the thyroid right lobe				
10.	Palpated the left lobe, switch hand positions and repeat the procedure				
	Evaluation				
1.	Compared findings with normal assessment				
2.	Identified unexpected outcomes				
3.	Recorded observation in nurses notes				
4.	Reported abnormalities to physician immediately				

Signature of Student ---------------------------------------

Signature of Clinical Instructor ------------------------------

Performance Evaluation: Gastric Lavage/Stomach Wash

Definition

Gastric lavage is the aspiration of the stomach contents and washing out of the stomach by means of a gastric tube.

Purpose

1. To obtain a specimen of gastric contents for diagnostic purpose.
2. To remove harmful substance swallowed accidentally or deliberately.
3. To cleans the stomach before endoscopic procedure.

Note: Physicians are required to carry out this procedure on unconscious patients. Specially credentialed nurse may carry it out on conscious patients. Two nurses are required to accomplish this procedure.

Equipment

1. Clean Trolley
2. Patient Trolley/ Bed table with head – down tilt mechanism
3. Suction apparatus
4. Oxygen supply
5. Stethoscope
6. Protective covering for the patient and the nurse
7. Clean patient gown
8. Sterile gloves
9. Denture container (as required)
10. Large bore orogastric tube
11. Large irrigating syringe
12. Funnel
13. Water – soluble lubricant
14. Bucket for aspirate
15. Gauze 12 swabs
16. Tape
17. Tap water (37°C) or appropriate antidote
18. Measuring jug
19. Mouth gag (if required)
20. Nasotracheal or endotracheal tubes with inflatable
21. Cuff (if required)
22. Sterile containers appropriately labelled for specimens of aspirate
23. Laboratory forms
24. Specimen bag for transpiration
25. Receptacle for soiled disposables.

Performance Phase: Procedure

Sl. No.	Performance Criteria	S	U	NP	Comments
	Assessment				
1.	Identified the client, explained procedure to the client				
2.	Ensured the patient's privacy				
3.	Determined client level of consciousness				
4.	Collected and arranged the equipments required				
5.	Assisted the client into the position				
6.	Washed and dried hands				
7.	Measured and recorded vital signs				

Contd...

Contd...

Sl. No.	Performance Criteria	S	U	NP	Comments
8.	Removed dentures and inspected the oral cavity for loose teeth. Whilst removing any secretion prevent his tongue from falling back				
9.	Measured the distance between the bridge of the nose and the xiphoid process and mark length on the orogastric tube				
10.	Lubricated the patient throughout soluble lubricant				
11.	Observed the patient throughout this activity				
12.	Passed the tube via the oral/nasal route while keeping the patient's head in a neutral position. Pass the tube to the indicated mark. Never forced the catheter. After the lavage tube is passed, the head of the table is lowered. Have suction available				
13.	Tested that tube is in the stomach by either • Aspirating some of the stomach contents and performing the litmus test Blue litmus paper will turn red • Placing a stethoscope over the epigastrium and syringe 2-3 mL of air into the tube • Placing some water in a reciver and submerge the free end of the tube below water level as the patient exhales				
14.	Aspirated the stomach contents with a syringe attached to the tube before instilling water or antidote, Saved the specimen for analysis				
15.	Removed the syringe and attach the funnel to the tube Elevated funnel or syringe and instill 150–300 mL of solution per instillation				
16.	Lowerd the funnel and allow the gastric content to flow into bucket				
17.	Saved samples of first washing				
18.	Recorded fluid input and output throughout the procedure				
19.	Repeated lavage until return is relatively clear and no particulate matter is seen				
20.	At completion of the lavage: The stomach was left empty				

Contd...

Contd...

Sl. No.	Performance Criteria	S	U	NP	Comments
21.	Kept the head lower than the body, pinch the tubing and removed				
22.	Cleaned the client and ensured that he is left feeling as comfortable as possible				
23.	Documented this procedure appropriately, monitored after effects and reported abnormal findings				
24.	Dispatched labelled specimens to laboratory				
25.	Replaced the equipment safely				
26.	Washed hands				

Signature of Student ---------------------------------------

Signature of Clinical Instructor -------------------------------

CHAPTER

5

Performance Evaluation of Hygienic Needs

Performance Evaluation: Antiseptic Hand Washing

Sl. No.	Performance Criteria	S	U	NP	Comments
	Assessment				
1.	Removed all jewelry, such as rings, watches and bracelets etc.				
2.	Turned on the faucet or elbow/ foot operated tap to achieve a moderately forceful flow				
3.	Adjusted the water temperature to lukewarm				
4.	Allowed the water to run continuously throughout the procedure, not touched the faucets or any part of the sink at any time during the procedure.				
5.	Holded hands and forearms in a downward direction below the elbow level when rinsing as well as washing during the procedure				
6.	Used liquid soap (if soap is used stored dry in a soap dish)				
7.	Scrubbed each hand with the other to produce a generous lather, using both rotatory and back and forth rubbing motions				
8.	Cleaned each cuticle and under each finger nail while holding hand under running water, then rinsed well				
9.	Lathered and scrubbed each palm and the back of each hand using friction motions. Cleaned the interdigital spaces by interlacing fingers				
10.	Rinsed hands thoroughly, lathered each wrist and forearm, and rinsed each arm working from below the elbow towards the fingertips				

Contd...

Contd...

Sl. No.	Performance Criteria	S	U	NP	Comments
11.	Allowed excess water to drip off from the fingertips after the final rinse				
12.	Dried with a clean towel beginning at fingertips and progressing up to the upper forearm				
13.	Completely dried with a fresh paper towel/ other dry part of the towel				
14.	Turned off the tap after washing				

Signature of Student ---------------------------------------

Signature of Clinical Instructor -------------------------------

Performance Evaluation: Bed Bath

Sl. No.	Performance Criteria	S	U	NP	Comments
	Assessment				
1.	Explained procedure to the client, encouraged the client to participate in the procedure as much as possible				
2.	Collected and prepared the equipments				
3.	Draw the bed side screen, applied bed breakers				
4.	Offered bed pan and asked the client to empty the bladder				
	Nursing diagnosis				
1.	Altered comfort related to activities intolerance				
	Planning				
1.	Developed individualized goals based on nursing diagnosis				
	Implementation				
1.	Washed and dried hands				
2.	Assisted client in to a comfortable position				
3.	Removed excess bed linen and bed appliances, left client covered with sheet, given mouth wash				
4.	Assisted the client to remove clothing				

Contd...

Contd...

Sl. No.	Performance Criteria	S	U	NP	Comments
5.	Checked the temperature of the water and poured into basin (changed water frequently throughout the procedure)				
6.	Asked the client to test the water temperature by placing hand into basin				
7.	Using the wash cloth (without soap), wiped one eye from inner canthus. Rinsed the wash cloth and cleaned the other eye				
8.	Washed the client face, ears and neck. Rinsed wash cloth and removed excess soap from the face. Dried the area				
9.	Exposed the arm opposite to her, placed towel length wise under it. Washed arm, axilla using firm strokes, rinsed and dried the area				
10.	Placed towel on the bed next to the client hand, placed and immersed hand in basin and washed, rinse and dried, trim the nail				
11.	Repeated step for the other arm				
12.	Spread towel across the chest, folded bed sheet, bathing blanket down to the umbilicus level. Washed, rinsed and dried the chest, kept the chest covered with a towel in between washing and rinsing				
13.	Lowered the sheet blanket down to the level of the umbilicus. Placed towel over the chest, washed rinsed and dried the abdomen				
14.	Spread the sheet/bath blanket, exposed the leg opposite and placed towel under the leg. Washed, rinse and dried the leg from ankle to knee and knee to groin using firm stroke				
15.	Placed a basin near the foot, placed client foot in the basin. Supported the ankle and heel, washed rinsed and dried the area				
16.	Changed water. Placed the client on side position exposing back and buttocks. Other supporter assisted the client				
17.	Washed, rinsed and dried the back and buttocks, payed attention to the gluteal folds and inspected for any redness or skin odors. Given back care				

Contd...

Contd...

Sl. No.	Performance Criteria	S	U	NP	Comments
18.	Changed the water and discarded the wash cloth and towel after washing the gluteal area				
19.	Assisted the client to wash, rinse dry his pubic area, washed from the front of the perineal area to the back Assisted client with a clean gown				
20.	Protected the pillow with a towel and combed the hair				
21.	Changed bed linen				
22.	Ensured the client is left with as comfortable as possible				
23.	Cleaned and disposed off all equipment				
24.	Washed and dried hands				
	Recording				
1.	Recorded the procedure in nursing progress sheet				

Signature of Student --

Signature of Clinical Instructor --------------------------------

Performance Evaluation: Assisting a Helpless Client in Brushing Teeth

Sl. No.	Performance Criteria	S	U	NP	Comments
	Assessment				
1.	Explained procedure to the client. Washed hands and put on the disposable gloves				
2.	Assessed client ability to grasp and manipulate tooth brush				
3.	Kept equipment within easy reach, and raised the bed to comfortable working position, sidelying position				
	Nursing diagnosis				
1.	Self-care deficit related to illness				
	Planning				
1.	Developed individualized goals based on nursing diagnosis				

Contd...

Contd...

Sl. No.	Performance Criteria	S	U	NP	Comments
	Implementation				
1.	Placed towel over the client chest				
2.	Applied toothpaste over emesis basin, poured small amount of water over tooth paste				
3.	Cleaned surfaces of teeth by holding top of bristles parallel with teeth and brushing gently back and front. Brushed the sides of teeth by moving bristles back and forth				
4.	Assisted client hold brush at 45 degree angle and lightly brush over surfaces and sides of the tongue				
5.	Allowed client to gargle the mouth with mouth wash solution as desired				
6.	Allowed the client to rinse mouth thoroughly and spit into emesis basin				
7.	Assisted the client to rest in a comfortable position and removed emesis basin and lowered bed to original position				
8.	Discarded the used items, removed soiled gloves and return equipment to proper place after cleaning it				
9.	Washed hands				
	Recording				
1.	Recorded procedure and noted, condition of oral cavity in nurses notes				

Signature of Student ---------------------------------------

Signature of Clinical Instructor ------------------------------

Performance Evaluation: Shampooing the Hair of Bed Ridden Client

Sl. No.	Performance Criteria	S	U	NP	Comments
	Assessment				
1.	Assessed risk factors for contraindication for shampooing				
2.	Discussed restriction for positioning client				
3.	Assessed client routine hair care practices style and type of hair care products				

Contd...

Contd...

Sl. No.	Performance Criteria	S	U	NP	Comments
4.	Assessed condition of client hair and scalp, noted distribution of hair, degree of oilness, hair texture, abrasions in the scalp, lacerations, lesions areas of inflammation and presence of infection/infestation (lice, dandruff, round worm infestation)				
	Nursing diagnosis				
1.	Self-care deficit related to illness				
	Planning				
1.	Developed individualized goals based on nursing diagnosis				
	Implementation				
1.	Washed hands				
2.	Arranged the equipment in a convenient place and lowered side rail				
3.	Placed water proof pad under client's shoulder neck and head. Positioned client with head and shoulders at the top edge of bed. Placed plastic trough under client head and bucket at the end of trough				
4.	Placed rolled towel under client neck and bath towel across client shoulder				
5.	Plugged the ears with non absorbent cotton				
6.	Brushed and combed client hair				
7.	Obtained water at about 43–44°C (110°F)				
8.	Placed the face towel over eyes				
9.	Poured water slowly from water pitcher over hair until it is completely wet. Then rinsed hair with saline. Applied small amount of shampoo				
10.	Worked up lather with both hands by applying pressure with finger tips				
11.	Rinsed hair with water. Repeated rinsing hair until hair is free of soap				
12.	Wraped client head in a bath towel. Dried client face with face towel to protect eyes. Dried off moisture along the neck and shoulder				

Contd...

Contd...

Sl. No.	Performance Criteria	S	U	NP	Comments
13.	Dried client hair and scalp using a second towel				
14.	Combed hair to remove tangles and dried with a drier				
15.	Assisted client to a comfortable position and completed styling of hair				
16.	Returned equipment to its proper place. Discarded soiled linen in linen hamper				
	Evaluation				
1.	Inspected condition of hair				
2.	Asked client the feeling after wash				
	Recording and reporting				
1.	Recorded procedure and reported to in charge nurse related to condition of hair and scalp				

Signature of Student ---------------------------------------

Signature of Clinical Instructor ------------------------------

Performance Evaluation: Back Care/Back Rub

Sl. No.	Performance Criteria	S	U	NP	Comments
	Assessment				
1.	Assessed the client has risk factors for skin impairment				
2.	Explained to the client the purpose of back care				
3.	Provided screen around the bed				
4.	Raised the bed level to convenient working height and lowered the side rails				
	Nursing diagnosis				
1.	Ineffective health maintenance				
	Planning				
1.	Developed individualized goals based on nursing diagnosis				
2.	Removed the client gown, untied the back ties and slipped the back portion of the gown toward the shoulders				

Contd...

Contd...

Sl. No.	Performance Criteria	S	U	NP	Comments
3.	Positioned the client on his or her side with the back towards the nurse				
4.	Placed a moderate amount of lotion to the hands and smooth the lotion around the entire surface of the palms				
5.	Applied hands first to the sacral area, massaging in circular motion, stroke upward from buttocks, i.e. shoulder massage over scapulas with smooth stroke continued in one smooth stroke to upper arms and laterally along side the back, down to iliac crests, not allowed hands to leave client skin. Continued massage pattern for 3 minutes				
6.	Knead skin by grasping tissue between thumb and finger knead upward along one side of spine from buttocks to shoulders and around nape of neck stroked down ward toward sacram repeated along other side of back				
7.	End massage with long stroking movements and informed client ending of back rub				
8.	Wiped excess lotion from client back with a bath towel, retied gown helped client to a comfortable position				
9.	Removed soiled towel and washed hands				
	Recording and reporting				
1.	Recorded condition of client skin and response to back care in nursing notes				

Signature of Student --

Signature of Clinical Instructor -------------------------------

Performance Evaluation: Providing Oral Hygiene

Sl. No.	Performance Criteria	S	U	NP	Comments
	Assessment				
1.	Assessed condition of lips, teeth, buccal mucosa, gums, palate and tongue, with wearing disposable gloves				

Contd...

Contd...

Sl. No.	Performance Criteria	S	U	NP	Comments
2.	Checked presence of dental problems like, dental caries, gingivitis, halitosis, stomatitis				
3.	Assessed client oral hygiene practices, such as frequency of tooth brushing, type of toothpaste and dental checkup				
4.	Assessed client ability to grasp and manipulate tooth brush				
5.	Arranged equipment at bed table				
	Nursing diagnosis				
1.	Ineffective health maintenance				
	Planning				
1.	Developed individualized goals based on nursing diagnosis				
	Implementation				
1.	Explained procedure to client				
2.	Raised bed to comfortable position. Assisted client to move to working position				
3.	Placed towel over client chest				
4.	Applied tooth paste to brush. Holding brush over emesis basin. Poured small amount of water over tooth paste				
5.	Client holds brush at 45° angle and lightly brushed over surface and sides of tongue				
6.	Allowed client to rinse mouth thoroughly by taking several sips of water, swishing water across all tooth surfaces and spitting into emesis basin				
7.	Allowed client to gargle and rinse mouth with mouth wash as desired				
8.	Assisted in wiping client mouth				
9.	Assisted client to comfortable position, removed emesis basin and bedside table				
10.	Removed gloves and disposed in receptacle. Performed hand hygiene				
	Evaluation				
1.	Repositioned client comfortably raised side rails, returned bed to original position				

Contd...

Contd...

Sl. No.	Performance Criteria	S	U	NP	Comments
2.	Replaced equipment after cleaning				
3.	Enquired client for any discomfort of oral cavity				
	Recording and report				
1.	Recorded the procedure in nurses notes				
2.	Reported unusual findings to in charge nurse.				

Signature of Student --------------------------------------

Signature of Clinical Instructor ------------------------------

Performance Evaluation: Performing Mouth Care for an Unconscious or Debilitated Client

Sl. No.	Performance Criteria	S	U	NP	Comments
	Assessment				
1.	Explained procedure to client				
2.	Washed hands and wored disposable gloves				
3.	Tested for presence of gag reflex by placing tongue depressor				
4.	Inspected the condition of oral cavity				
	Nursing diagnosis				
1.	Ineffective health maintenance				
	Planning				
1.	Developed individualized goals based on nursing diagnosis				
	Implementation				
1.	Positioned client on side with head turned well toward dependent side				
2.	Arranged the equipment near the bed side				
3.	Provided curtain around the bed				
4.	Placed towel under client head and kidney tray under chin				
5.	Carefully separated and lowered teeth with padded tongue blade by inserting blade quickly but gently between the back molar, inserted when client relaxed without force				

Contd...

Contd...

Sl. No.	Performance Criteria	S	U	NP	Comments
6.	Cleaned mouth using cotton rolls fixed well in the artery forceps, moistened with water. Cleaned chewing and inner tooth surfaces first, then after tooth surfaces cheeks, gently swab tongue but avoided stimulating gag reflex. Then cleaned with swab wet with water, removed excess water from the swab by squeezing wet swab with forceps.				
7.	Suctioned secretion which accumulated				
8.	Applied thin layer of water soluble jelly to lip				
9.	Informed client that the procedure is completed				
10.	Removed gloves and disposed in receptacle				
	Evaluation				
1.	Repositioned client comfortably raised side rails, returned bed to original position				
2.	Replaced equipment after cleaning				
3.	Washed hands				
	Recording and reporting				
1.	Recorded the procedure. Noted presence of bleeding gums, dry mucous, ulceration, and crust on tongue				
2.	Reported unusual findings to in charge nurse.				

Signature of Student --

Signature of Clinical Instructor --------------------------------

Performance Evaluation: Performing Nail and Foot Care

Sl. No.	Performance Criteria	S	U	NP	Comments
	Assessment				
1.	Assessed all surfaces of fingers, toes, feet for dryness and inflammation				
2.	Assessed color and temperature of toes, feet and fingers				

Contd...

Contd...

Sl. No.	Performance Criteria	S	U	NP	Comments
3.	Discussed the history of foot or nail problem/ any systemic disease like diabetes, hypertension etc.				
4.	Discussed client regular practices for care of nail and foot				
	Nursing diagnosis				
1.	Ineffective health maintenance				
	Planning				
1.	Developed individualized goals based on nursing diagnosis				
	Implementation				
1.	Explained procedure to client				
2.	Collected articles required, arranged over bed table				
3.	Positioned the client in a bed side chair				
4.	Filled washbasin with warm water. Tested water temperature (43–44° centigrade)				
5.	Instructed the client to place feet in basin for soaking toe nails				
6.	Allowed the client feet to soak for 10 minutes				
7.	Clipped toe nail straight across using nail clipper				
8.	Removed feet from basin and dried thoroughly				
9.	Wiped each toe nail with dry cloth, applied lotion to toenails				
10.	Instructed client to place fingers in basin, over bed table for soaking finger nails				
11.	Clipped fingers nails straight across, using nail clipper, shaped nails with file				
12.	Moved over bed table away from client				
13.	Applied lotion to fingers and hands and helped client to back to bed into comfortable position				
	Evaluation				
1.	Removed disposable gloves and replaced equipments				

Contd...

Contd...

Sl. No.	Performance Criteria	S	U	NP	Comments
2.	Inspected nails and surrounding skin surfaces				
3.	Recorded procedure and observation in nurses notes				
4.	Reported significance of nail and surrounding condition to charge nurse				

Signature of Student --

Signature of Clinical Instructor --------------------------------

Performance Evaluation: Perineal Care (Male and Female)

Sl. No.	Performance Criteria	S	U	NP	Comments
	Assessment				
1.	Identified clients risk for developing infection of genetalia				
2.	Discussed client knowledge of perineal hygienc				
	Nursing diagnosis				
1.	Ineffective health maintenance				
	Planning				
1.	Developed individualized goals based on nursing diagnosis				
	Implementation				
1.	Explained procedure and its purpose to client				
2.	Prepared needed equipment and supplies				
3.	Assisted client to assuming side lying position, placed towel length wise, keeping client covered with sheet				
4.	Applied disposable gloves				
5.	Cleansed buttock and anus washing front to back and dried area thoroughly				
6.	Changed gloves when they are soiled, performed hand hygiene				
7.	Folded top bed linen down toward foot of bed and raise client gown above genital area, protected client privacy				
8.	Placed wash basin, wash cloth and toilet tissue on over bed table				

Contd...

Contd...

Sl. No.	Performance Criteria	S	U	NP	Comments
	Female perineal care				
1.	Assisted client to dorsal recumbent position				
2.	Lowered side rail, and helped client to flex knees and spread legs				
3.	Washed and dried client upper thighs				
4.	Washed labia majora. Washed carefully the skin folds. Wiped in direction from perineum to rectum (front to back)				
5.	Separated labia, exposed urethral and vaginal orifice with dominant hand, washed down from pubic area toward rectum. Used separate section of cloth for each stroke				
6.	Placed bed pan under the client's buttock, poured warm water over perineal area. Dried perineal area thoroughly using front to back method				
7.	Instructed client to lower legs and assume comfortable position				
	Male perineal care				
1.	Lowered side rails and assisted client to supine position				
2.	Washed and dried client upper thighs				
3.	Gently raised penis, and placed bath towel underneath. Gently grasped shaft of penis				
4.	Washed tip of penis at urethral meatus. First using circular motion, clensed from meatus outward. Discarded wash cloth until penis is clean. Rinse and dried gently				
5.	Returned foreskin to its natural position				
6.	Washed shaft of penis with gentle downward strokes, instructed client to spread legs apart slightly				
7.	Gently cleansed scrotum lifted carefully and washed underlying skin folds				
8.	Assisted client to turning side lying position				
9.	Removed disposable gloves				
	Evaluation				
1.	Assisted client in assuming comfortable position and covered with sheet				

Contd...

Contd...

Sl. No.	Performance Criteria	S	U	NP	Comments
2.	Inspected surface of external genitalia and surrounding skin after cleansing				
	Record and report				
1.	Recorded procedure in nursing notes				
2.	Reported observation to charge nurse				

Signature of Student ---------------------------------------

Signature of Clinical Instructor -------------------------------

CHAPTER

6

Performance Evaluation of Nutrition Aspect

Performance Evaluation: Performing Nutritional Assessment

Nutritional assessment is a specific, measurable means of identifying clients who may be malnourished. Clients may be assessed for a variety of reasons, including having diagnosis associated with nutrition problems (such as burns or malabsorption) recent rapid weight loss, or history of poor dietary intake.

Sl. No.	Performance Criteria	S	U	NP	Comments
	Assessment				
1.	Determined need to perform nutritional assessment based on diagnosis and history				
2.	Assessed client body weight				
3.	Reviewed results of laboratory tests				
	Nursing Diagnosis				
1.	Altered nutrition, less than body requirements, related factors based on client assessment data				
	Planning				
1.	Client will understand purpose of nutritional assessment and its effect on health care				
	Implementation				
1.	Explained procedure to client				
2.	Obtained complete and thorough nursing history and performed physical assessment				
3.	Assisted client to stand on weighing scale and recorded weight				
4.	Measured client height using measuring tape				
5.	Measured mid arm circumference at midpoint of arm in centimeters (between tip of acromial process of scapula and olecranon process of ulna) and recorded				

Contd...

Contd...

Sl. No.	Performance Criteria	S	U	NP	Comments
6.	Skin fold measurements are used to estimate fat content of subcutaneous tissue				
7.	Assisted client to comfortable position				
8.	Washed hands				
9.	Explained client that nutritional assessment is completed				
	Evaluation				
1.	Compared client height, weight, midarm circumference with normal measurement				
	Recording and reporting				
1.	Recorded results on nutritional assessment form				
2.	Reported significant difference to in charge nurse				

Signature of Student ---------------------------------------

Signature of Clinical Instructor ------------------------------

Performance Evaluation: Feeding a Helpless Client

Assisting the adult for feeding (eating). Oral nutrition requires time, patience, knowledge and understanding. Most people eat without assistance. However with illness or trauma the client may be physically unable to eat without assistance. Physical impairments that limit self feeding include hemiplegia, fractured arm, and quadriplegia, debilitating illness, or generalized weakness. The presence of intravenous therapy, dressings can also limit self feeding. Also, some older adults tire quickly and may need to be assisted even they can eat independently. Although, adult feeding needs and techniques differ from those for infants. The adult who needs help to eat still needs compassion and understanding. Merely feeding the adult can be accomplished with common sense, but providing a socially meaningful mealtime requires education and experience on the part of the nurse.

Sl .No.	Performance Criteria	S	U	NP	Comments
	Assessment				
1.	Assessed the client what type of diet he can tolerate				
2.	Assessed client ability to swallow				
3.	Determined the ability of client in self feed				
4.	Assessed client appetite, tolerance to food, likes and dislikes				
	Nursing Diagnosis				
1.	Feeding self care deficit				
	Planning				
1.	Develop individualized goals for the clients based on the nursing diagnosis. Client will participate in feeding • Prepare client for meal • Help client urinate or defecate • Help client to wash hands • Assist client to comfortable sitting position • Obtain special devices and needed supplies to facilitate feeding				
	Implementation				
1.	Washed hands before preparing client tray				
2.	Prepared tray to meet clients needs				
3.	Asked the client about his like to eat, and cut food into bite sized pieces				
4.	Fed the client in a manner that facilitates chewing and swallowing. Assessed chewing and swallowing				
5.	Provided fluids as required, talked to client during meal				
6.	Not allowed client to drink all liquids at beginning of meal				
7.	During feeding given health education regarding nutrition				
8.	Assisted client to wash hands and performed mouth care				
9.	Assisted client to resting position				
	Evaluation				
1.	During meal noted client ability to swallow				

Contd...

Contd...

Sl .No.	Performance Criteria	S	U	NP	Comments
	Recording and reporting				
1.	Documented client tolerance of diet, amount eaten, intake and output				
2.	Reported to charge nurse regarding feeding of client				

Signature of Student -------------------------------------

Signature of Clinical Instructor -----------------------------

Performance Evaluation—Insertion of Nasogastric Tube (Small Bore for Enteral Feeding)

When the client is unable to ingest food enteral tube feeding is indicated. Feeding tube can be inserted through the nose (Nasogastric) complication associated with tube feeding. Small bore feeding tubes create less discomfort for the client and currently most often used.

Sl. No.	Performance Criteria	S	U	NP	Comments
	Assessment				
1.	Assessed client for need of nasogastric intubation				
2.	Identified the client				
3.	Reviewed client medical history for nasal problems				
4.	Reviewed physician order for type of tube				
5.	Predetermined a signal by which the client can communicate if he requires the nurse to halt the procedure, e.g. raise his hands				
	Nursing diagnosis				
1.	Self care deficit, feeding (oral nutrition)				
	Planning				
1.	Client will be able to maintain normal nutrition and fluid level				
	Implementation				
1.	Performed hand hygiene				

Contd...

Contd...

Sl. No.	Performance Criteria	S	U	NP	Comments
2.	Explained procedure to client and assisted client to high fowlers position				
3.	Placed bath towel over chest				
4.	Established the distance that the tube is to be passed by measuring the distance on the tube from the client ear lobe to the bridge of the nose to the bottom of the xiphisternum				
5.	Determined length of tube to be inserted and mark with tape				
6.	Used clean technique to assess the equipment				
7.	Cut tape 10 cm (4 m inches) long for tube fixing				
8.	Lubricated about 15–20 cm of the tube with water soluble jelly, which has been placed on a gauze swab				
9.	Asked client to relax as much as possible while the tube is passed				
10.	Inserted the tube and slide it gently but firmly inwards and backwards along the floor of the nose to the nasopharynx				
11.	Encouraged client to swallow and breath through his mouth when the tube reaches the pharynx keeping the chin down head forward to assist the passage of the tube				
12.	Advanced the tube until the length previously measured has been inserted and mark has reached the external nares				
13.	Ascertained whether the tube is in the stomach • Aspirated the contents of the stomach with a syringe and done the litmus test (blue litmus paper should turn to red). • Placed the stethoscope over the epigastrium and inject 2–3 mL of air to the tube and detected air whooshing sounds				
14.	Aspirated the stomach contents as per instruction. Dispatched specimen to laboratory				
15.	Secured the tube to the client nose with tape. Secured the free end of the tube in the suitable position avoiding visual obstruction				

Contd...

Contd...

Sl. No.	Performance Criteria	S	U	NP	Comments
	Evaluation				
1.	Ensured that the client is left feeling as comfortable as possible				
2.	Cleaned and disposed the equipments				
3.	Observed client for any difficulty in breathing, coughing or gagging				
4.	Washed hands				
5.	Monitored the after effects				
	Recording and reporting				
1.	Documented the nursing procedure in nursing chart				
2.	Recorded intake and output chart				

Signature of Student ---------------------------------------

Signature of Clinical Instructor -------------------------------

Performance Evaluation: Administering Tube Feeding

Administration of enteral tube feeding via Nasogastric tube is a nursing procedure. Feeding will be initiated after tube placement verified.

Sl. No.	Performance Criteria	S	U	NP	Comments
	Assessment				
1.	Assessed client need for tube feeding				
2.	Auscultate for bowel sounds before feeding				
	Nursing diagnosis				
1.	Self care deficit, feeding (oral nutrition)				
	Planning				
1.	Client will be able to maintain normal nutrition and fluid level				
2.	Explained procedure to the client				
3.	Prepared feeding container to administer, and prepared planned food content to tube feeding at room temperature				
4.	For intermittent feeding kept syringe ready				

Contd...

Contd...

Sl. No.	Performance Criteria	S	U	NP	Comments
	Implementation				
1.	Checked placement of tube by means of aspiration of gastric juice is by checking with stethoscope while introducing air in to the stomach				
2.	Positioned the client to high fowlers position				
3.	Placed a towel under the chin				
4.	Examined the appearance of aspirated contents by Ph testing				
5.	Flushed tubing with water				
6.	Pinched proximal end of the feeding tube and elevated to 18 inches above the client head. Filled syringe with the required feed, allowed syringe to empty gradually. Refilled the prescribed amount has been given to the client				
6.	Rinse tube with water				
7.	Rinse the tube with plain water at the end of feeding				
8.	Washed hands				
	Evaluation				
1.	When gastric residual exceeds 100 mL, stop feeding, inform physician				
2.	Client develops nausea and vomiting inform physician				
	Recording and reporting				
1.	Recorded amount of feeding, client response to tube feeding and untoward effects in nurses notes				
2.	Recorded intake and output				

Signature of Student ---------------------------------------

Signature of Clinical Instructor -------------------------------

CHAPTER

7

Performance Evaluation of Elimination

Performance Evaluation: Collecting Stool Specimen

Laboratory examination and analysis of stool provides useful information about the nature of elimination. Stool specimens are collected to determine pathologic conditions such as tumors, hemorrhage, infection and malabsorption problems. These conditions can be detected by the presence of blood, bile, urobilinogen, fat, nitrogen content, ova, parasites, protozoa, and bacteria. Single stool specimens are most frequently collected. But occasionally stool is collected for a timed period such as 72 hours.

Sl. No.	Performance Criteria	S	U	NP	Comments
	Assessment				
1.	Determined purpose of stool specimen and correct method of handling specimen				
2.	Explained to client that modification and restriction of food as per desired investigation				
3.	Discussed normal defecation pattern of client				
4.	Assessed client for gastrointestinal dysfunction, such as abdominal pain, nausea, vomiting, excessive flatus etc.				
5.	Assessed ability to assist in collection of stool specimen • ability to use toilet facilities • ability to handle specimen container				
	Nursing diagnosis				
1.	• Bowel incontinence • Toileting self care deficit				
	Planning				
1.	Developed individualized goals for the client based on nursing diagnosis				
2.	Explained reason for collection of stool specimen to client				

Contd...

Contd...

Sl. No.	Performance Criteria	S	U	NP	Comments
	Implementation				
1.	Assessed client the need of bed pan. Instructed client to void before defecating (discard urine before collecting specimen in bedpan)				
2.	Provided client with clean, dry, bedpan and specimen container potty chair in which to defecate				
3.	Instructed client to wash after toileting				
4.	Put on clean disposable gloves				
5.	Obtained specimen and transferred to proper container				
6.	Washed hands				
7.	Attached specimen identification label and laboratory requisition with date time test name on it				
8.	Sent specimen to laboratory immediately				
	Evaluation				
1.	Noted character of stool with normal laboratory values				
2.	Compared client laboratory test results with normal laboratory values				
	Recording and reporting				
1.	Recorded time and date specimen collected and dispositions in nurses notes				
2.	Recorded appearance and odor of stool				
3.	Informed result to physician				

Signature of Student -------------------------------------

Signature of Clinical Instructor -----------------------------

Performance Evaluation: Administering an Enema

An enema is the instillation of a solution into the rectum and sigmoid colon. The primary reason for an enema is promotion of defecation by stimulating peristalisis. The volume and type of fluid instilled break up the fecal mass, stretches the rectal wall, and initiates the defecation reflex. Clients should not rely on enemas to maintain bowel regularity because they do not treat the cause of irregularity or constipation. Frequent enemas disrupt normal defecation reflexes, resulting in independence on enemas for elimination.

Sl. No.	Performance Criteria	S	U	NP	Comments
	Assessment				
1.	Assessed status of client last bowel movement, level of awareness, normal bowel patterns, hemorrhoids, mobility, external sphincter control, abdominal pain				
2.	Determined clients level of understanding of purpose of enema				
3.	Checked client medical record to clarify the rationale for the enema				
	Nursing diagnosis				
1.	• Constipation • Pain				
	Planning				
1.	Developed individualized goals for the client based on nursing diagnosis • Client immediate constipation will be relieved • Client will be free of fecal impaction • Bowel will be adequately cleansed in preparation for a diagnostic or surgical procedure				
	Implementation				
1.	Washed hands and applied gloves				
2.	Provided privacy by closing curtains around bed				
3.	Raised bed to appropriate height and raised side rail on opposite side				
4.	Assisted client in to left side lying (Sim's) position with right knee flexed. Positioned client on bed pan in comfortable dorsal recumbent position				
5.	Placed waterproof pad under hips and buttocks				
6.	Covered client with bath blanket, exposing only rectal area, clearly visualizing anus				
7.	Placed bed pan in easily accessible position				

Contd...

Contd...

Sl. No.	Performance Criteria	S	U	NP	Comments
8.	Administered enema using prepackaged disposable container • Removed plastic cap from rectal tip. Tip is already lubricated but more jelly can be applied as needed • Gently separated buttocks to locate rectum, instruct client to relax by breathing out slowly through mouth • Inserted tip of bottle tube gently into rectum (adult - 7.5 to 10 cm (3–4 inches), Child - 5 to 7.5 cm (2–3 inches), Infant - 2.5 to 3.7 cm (1–1.5 inches).				
9.	Squeezed bottle until all of solution has entered into rectum and colon (most bottle contain approximately 250 mL of solution)				
10.	Placed layers of toilet tissue around tube at anus and gently withdraw rectal tube				
11.	Assessed the client to find the feeling of distention is normal. Asked client to retain solution as long as possible while lying quietly in bed				
12.	Discard enema container and tubing in proper receptacle				
13.	Assisted client to position on bed pan				
14.	Observed character of feces and solution				
15.	Assisted client as needed to wash anal area with soap and warm water				
16.	Removed gloves and discarded and washed hands				
	Evaluation				
1.	Inspected color, consistency, amount of stool and the amount of fluid passed				
2.	Assessed condition of abdomen				
	Recording and reporting				
1.	Recorded type and volume of enema given and the results				
2.	Reported result of enema to physician				

Signature of Student -------------------------------------

Signature of Clinical Instructor ------------------------------

Performance Evaluation: Urinary Catheterization

Definition

Urinary catheterization is the insertion of a catheter into the bladder, using aseptic technique, for the purpose of evacuating or instilling fluids.

Purpose

1. To empty the contents of the bladder, e.g. before or after abdominal, pelvic or rectal surgery and before certain investigations.
2. To determine residual urine.
3. To allow bladder irrigation.
4. To bypass an obstruction.
5. To relieve retention of urine and incontinence.
6. To introduce cytotoxic drugs in the treatment of papillary bladder carcinoma.
7. To perform bladder function tests.
8. To measure urinary output accurately.

In the female, urinary catheterization may be carried out for the eight reasons listed above and for the two further reason:

Equipment

1. Clean trolley
2. Sterile catheterization pack containing forceps, receiver, gauze swabs.
3. Lubricant
4. Disposable pad
5. Sterile gloves
6. Appropriate sterile urinary catheter
7. Antiseptic solution or normal saline
8. Sterile container for analysis if required
9. Standing lamp if available
10. Drainage bag
11. Hypoallergenic tape

Procedure

Male

Sl. No.	Performance Criteria	S	U	NP	Comments
	Assessment				
1.	Checked the physician's order, progress notes, and nursing care plan				
2.	Identified the client				
3.	Explained the procedure to the patient				
4.	Ensured privacy				
5.	Assisted the patient to get into supine position with knees bent. Do not expose the genital area at this stage				
6.	Directed the standing lamp (if available) For visualization of genital area				
7.	Washed and dried hands				
8.	Opened sterile catheterization package and sterile catheter using aseptic technique				
9.	Placed disposable pad across the patient's thighs and under buttocks				
10.	Do not sterile gloves				
11.	Applied lubricant to the nozzle of the catheter				

Female

1.	Separated the labia minora so that the urethral meatus is visualized. One hand is to maintain separation of the labia until catheterization is finished				
2.	Cleans around the urethral meatus with normal saline or antiseptic solution. Manipulated cleansing sponges with forceps, cleansing with downward strokes. Dispose of sponge after each use				
3.	Handled the tip of the catheter, placing its end in the receiver between the patient's legs				
4.	Introduced the well lubricated tip of the catheter into the urethral meatus using strict aseptic technique. Inserted catheter in an upward and backward direction for 5–7 cm (2–3 inches). Avoided contaminating surface of catheter				

Contd...

Contd...

5.	Allowed some bladder urine to flow through catheter before connecting the bag				
6.	Inflated the balloon according to the manufacture's instructions, having ensured that the catheter is draining adequately				

Male

7.	Washed off penis around urinary meatus with normal saline / antiseptic solution. Cleanse urethral meatus from tip to foreskin with downward stroke. Dispose sponge after each use. Keep the foreskin retracted. Maintain sterility of dominant hand.				
8.	Grasped shaft of penis and elevate it. Insert catheter into the urethra applying gentle traction to penis while catheter is passed				
9.	Advanced catheter 15–25 cm (6–10 inches)				
10.	Inflated the balloon according to the manufacturer's instructions				
11.	Withdrawn the catheter slightly and connect to the drainage system				
12.	Anchored the catheter by taping laterally				
13.	Dried area. Position the patient comfortably				
14.	Measure the amount of urine				
15.	Disposed of equipment as appropriate				
16.	Washed and dried hands (refer to Hand Washing procedure)				
17.	Documented the procedure appropriately. Recorded date and time, type of catheter used and size, color and amount of urine, client tolerance, and any other relevant observations				

Signature of Student --------------------------------------

Signature of Clinical Instructor ------------------------------

Performance Evaluation: Inserting Rectal Tube

A rectal tube is occasionally aid in the relief of abdominal distention secondary to unexcelled flatus. Such distention frequently occurs after abdominal

surgery. The tube may remain in place for several minute to allow flatus to escape.

Sl. No.	Performance Criteria	S	U	NP	Comments
	Assessment				
1.	Assessed patient for abdominal distention, amount of flatus patient is passing, existing pathologic condition related to intestinal disorders, bowel sounds etc.				
2.	Checked physician order for specific instructions in use of rectal tube				
	Nursing diagnosis				
1.	Pain—related to factors based on a patient condition or needs				
	Planning				
1.	Patient will experience relief, distention is relieved Patient will experience a reduction in abdominal distention				
	Implementation				
1.	Washed hands and applied gloves				
2.	Provided privacy				
3.	Raised bed to appropriate height				
4.	Asked patient to turn into left side and assume side lying or Sims position, kept patient draped except for rectal area				
5.	Placed water proof pad under buttocks				
6.	Lubricated tip of rectal tube generously				
7.	Taken care to expose patient minimally. Gently separate buttocks, locate anus, and ask patient to take deep breath and slowly exhale through mouth				
8.	Inserted tip of rectal tube slowly, pointing it in direction of umbilicus, ensuring that tube in place (Tube can be inserted to adult up to 15 cm (6")				
9.	After inserting tube, tape it to lower buttock				
10.	Allowed rectal tube to remain in place for no longer than 30 minutes				

Contd...

Contd...

Sl. No.	Performance Criteria	S	U	NP	Comments
11.	Removed gloves and wash hands after leaving bedside and before removing rectal tube				
12.	Remove rectal tube with gloved hands and cleaned client rectal area				
13.	Returned patient to comfortable position				
	Evaluation				
1.	Palpated patients abdomen for firmness and distention				
2.	Asked patient if relief was obtained from rectal tube				
	Recording and reporting				
1.	Recorded procedure in nurses progress notes and reported physical assessment findings before and after procedure and tube insertion				

Signature of Student ---------------------------------------

Signature of Clinical Instructor -------------------------------.

Performance Evaluation: Care of Urethral Catheter

Sl. No.	Performance Criteria	S	U	NP	Comments
	Assessment				
1.	Identifies the client with urethral catheter				
2.	Assembles necessary equipment				
	Implementation				
1.	Tapes the catheter of male client to the abdomen				
2.	Tapes the catheter to female clients to the inner thigh				
3.	Ensures that a closed system maintained between the the catheter and the drainage bag				
4.	Maintains urinary drainage bag in a dependent position				

Contd...

Contd...

Sl. No.	Performance Criteria	S	U	NP	Comments
5.	Performed catheter care with antiseptic solution and water every 24 hours				
6.	Retract foreskin on uncircumcised male client to perform catheter care and returns foreskin over the glans when catheter care is completed				
7.	Irrigates the catheter only as needed with normal saline or acid citrate solution (exception bladder trauma or surgery)				
8.	Changes the catheter when sediment adheres to the drainage tubing when the catheter is obstructed or when the catheter leaks				
9.	Obtains urine specimen as needed for diagnosis studies while maintaining a closed system				
	Recording and reporting				
1.	Recorded procedure in nursing notes				
2.	Reported to charge nurse about care provided				

Signature of Student ---------------------------------------

Signature of Clinical Instructor -------------------------------

Performance Evaluation: Care of Suprapubic Catheter

Sl. No.	Performance Criteria	S	U	NP	Comments
	Assessment				
1.	Identifies the client with suprapubic catheter				
2.	Observes for signs of hemorrhage and peritonitis				
	Implementation				
1.	Changes the dressing daily, inspecting the insertion site, and maintains a dry, sterile dressing				
2.	Maintains the drainage system				

Contd...

Contd...

Sl. No.	Performance Criteria	S	U	NP	Comments
3.	Ensures that the catheter is sutured and taped securely to the client				
4.	Maintains the drainage bag in a dependent position				
5.	Obtains urine specimen maintaining a closed system				
6.	Observes catheter clamping protocol as ordered				
	Recording and reporting				
1.	Records superpubic catheter output separately from other urinary output measurement				
2.	Documents all pertinent information in nurses notes				
3.	Inform significant changes to physician				
4.	Reported to charge nurse about care provided				

Signature of Student --------------------------------------

Signature of Clinical Instructor -------------------------

Performance Evaluation: Measuring and Recording Intake and Output

Sl. No.	Performance Criteria	S	U	NP	Comments
	Assessment				
1.	Reviewed indication for intake and output				
2.	Reviewed history of • Fever, wound infection • Gastric suction • IV infusion • Chest or abdominal surgery • Burns, hemodynamic monitoring • Patient on diuretics, steroids • Head injury or any other trauma • Endocrine imbalance • Diabetic keto acidosis etc.				
3.	Observed the signs of dehydration/over hydration				
4.	Inspected urine color and specific gravity				

Contd...

Contd...

Sl. No.	Performance Criteria	S	U	NP	Comments
	Nursing diagnosis				
1.	• Fluid volume deficit • Fluid volume excess				
	Planning				
1.	• The client will maintain a minimum of 1500 oral intake per 24 hours • Client physical assessment and laboratory values will return to, and remain within normal limit				
	Implementation				
1.	Explained the client and family the importance of intake and output measurement to their client				
2.	Measured and recorded all fluids taken by mouth • Liquids with meals • Liquid taken with medication • Parenteral fluids • Enteral tube feeding				
3.	Measured and Recorded urine output, drainage bag collection, bed pan collection etc.				
4.	Removed gloves, washed hands after measuring and recording output fluids				
	Evaluation				
1.	Inspected client's fluid status as per assessment. Evaluated condition of skin and tissue				
2.	Observed color of urine				
3.	Noted intake and output balance				
	Recording and reporting				
1.	Calculated total intake and output and recorded with all features and reported to in charge nurse				

Signature of Student ---------------------------------------

Signature of Clinical Instructor -------------------------------

CHAPTER

8

Performance Evaluation of Specimen Collection

Nurses often assume responsibility for collection of specimen of body secretion and excretion. Laboratory examination of specimen of urine, stool, sputum, blood and wound drainage provides important information of body functioning and contributes to the assessment of health status. Laboratory test results can facilitate diagnosis of health problems, provide information about the stage and activity of a disease process, and measures the response to therapy.

Performance Evaluation: Collecting a Random Urine Specimen

Urine is the most frequently collected specimen because its examination provides valuable clues about functioning of the human body. A urinary analysis can provides information about the status of kidney function, nutrition, metabolic function, and certain systemic diseases. Urine collection is part of every clients testing when admitted to a healthcare facility.

Procedure

Sl. No.	Performance Criteria	S	U	NP	Comments
	Assessment				
1.	Assessed client ability to provide specimen independently. Able to position self, hold container, stand or sit to void				
2.	Assessed for signs and symptoms of urinary tract infection, frequency, urgency, dysuria, hematuria, flank pain, fever, cloudy urine with sediments, foul odor etc.				
	Nursing diagnosis				
1.	Ineffective coping related to specimen collection				
	Planning				
1.	Client will be able to collect urine specimen without contamination				

Contd...

Contd...

Sl. No.	Performance Criteria	S	U	NP	Comments
	Implementation				
1.	Washed hands and prepared equipment at bed side				
2.	Provided towel, wash cloth, to cleanse perineal area				
3.	Given specimen container and directed to bathroom. Assisted client as needed to void into specimen container				
4.	Placed lid tightly on container without touching inside the lid				
5.	Washed it off outside of container (for splashed urine)				
6.	Removed and discarded gloves and washed hands				
7.	Securely attached properly completed identification label and laboratory requisition to specimen				
8.	Sent specimen to laboratory immediately				
	Evaluation				
1.	Compared results of client urinanalysis with normal laboratory values				
	Recording and reporting				
1.	Recorded collection of specimen in nurses notes, noted time, date, purpose, appearance and odor of urine				
2.	Reported to physician, significant abnormalities				

Signature of Student --

Signature of Clinical Instructor --------------------------------

Performance Evaluation: Culture and Sensitivity Test (Clean Voided) Urine Specimen

A common test performed on urine is a culture and sensitivity measurement. A few drops of urine are placed on a special medium to determine if bacteria are present. Reading are made at 24 and 48 hours intervals and the final reading is made after 72 hours. If bacteria are present, sensitivity testing reveals the antibiotics that will be effective against the microorganisms.

Procedure

Sl. No.	Performance Criteria	S	U	NP	Comments
	Assessment				
1.	Assessed client mobility and balance in being able to use toilet facilities independently				
2.	Assessed risk factors for urinary tract infection				
3.	Assessed purpose of test and method of collection				
	Nursing diagnosis				
1.	Ineffective management regarding specimen collection				
	Planning				
1.	Client able to collect urine specimen without contamination				
2.	Client able to collect urine specimen free of feces				
	Implementation				
1.	Provided privacy for client by closing curtain around bed				
2.	Provided client towel, wash cloth to cleanse perineum				
3.	Assisted bedridden client into bedpan				
4.	Do not sterile gloves				
5.	Opened specimen container and placed cap with sterile inside surface up without touching inside of container				
6.	Assisted client to independently cleanse perineum and collect specimen				
7.	After client has initiated urine stream, pass urine				
8.	Removed specimen container before flow of urine. Client finishes voiding in to bedpan				
9.	Replaced cap securely on specimen container				
10.	Cleansed urine from exterior surface of container				

Contd...

Contd...

Sl. No.	Performance Criteria	S	U	NP	Comments
11.	Disposed of bed pan, remove and discard gloves and wash hands				
12.	Labeled specimen and attach laboratory requisition				
13.	Taken specimen to laboratory within 15 minutes				
	Evaluation				
1.	Assessed client urine culture and sensitivity report for bacterial growth				
	Recording and reporting				
1.	Recorded date and time urine specimen was obtained in nurses notes				
2.	Reported to physician about laboratory result				

Signature of Student ---------------------------------------

Signature of Clinical Instructor -------------------------------

Performance Evaluation: Collecting a Timed Urine Specimen

Some tests of renal function and urine composition require urine to be collected over 2, to 72 hours. The 24 hours timed collection is most common. The tests allow for the measurement of elements such as amino acids, creatinine, hormones, glucose and adrenocorticosteroids, whose levels change over time. Timed collections can also provide a means to measure the concentration or dilution of urine.

Timed urine collections begin after a client urinates. The nurse discards the first specimen and then collects every successive specimen until the timed period has ended. Each specimen is transferred immediately to a large collection bottle kept in the client bathroom. Any missed specimens make test result inaccurate. The client should always void the last specimen as close as possible to the end of the collection period.

Procedure

Sl. No.	Performance Criteria	S	U	NP	Comments
	Assessment				
1.	Determined purpose of timed urine specimen collection				
2.	Assessed client ability to collect specimens independently				
	Nursing diagnosis				
1.	Ineffective management regarding specimen collection				
	Planning				
1.	Client will be able to collect urine specimen without contamination				
	Implementation				
1.	Provided privacy for client by closing curtain around bed				
2.	Provided client towel, wash cloth to cleanse perineum				
3.	Applied gloves when handling urine				
4.	Discarded first specimen as test begins and recorded time test begins on laboratory requisition form				
5.	Advised client to have water as required				
6.	Placed signs indicating timed urine specimen on client bed, on urinal, bedpan. specimen container				
7.	Measured volume of each voiding				
8.	Placed all voided urine into labeled specimen container				
9.	Washed hands and discarded gloves after collection of each voiding				
10.	Instructed the client to drink two glass of water 1 hour before timed urine collection ends				
11.	Encouraged client to drink two glasses of water 1 hour before timed urine collection ends				
12.	Encouraged client to empty bladder during last 15 minutes of urine collection period				

Contd...

Contd...

Sl. No.	Performance Criteria	S	U	NP	Comments
13.	At end of period sent labeled specimen to laboratory with appropriate requisition				
	Evaluation				
1.	Assessed client urine report with normal laboratory values				
2.	Removed room signs after specimen collection				
	Recording and reporting				
1.	Recorded starting time of urine collection in nurses notes				
2.	At completion of test, recorded the time urine collection is finished, the appearance, amount and odor of the urine				
3.	Discussed abnormal test result with physician				

Signature of Student --------------------------------------

Signature of Clinical Instructor ------------------------------

Performance Evaluation: Collecting a Sterile Urine Specimen from an Indwelling Catheter

It is often necessary to collect urine specimens from a client who has an indwelling catheter. Strict aseptic technique should be used to ensure sterility and to avoid introducing infection into the urinary tract.

A urine specimen should not be collected for culture tests from a urine drainage bag unless it is the first urine to drain into a new sterile bag. Bacteria grow rapidly in drainage bags and can give a false measurement of bacteria in the urine.

Procedure

Sl. No.	Performance Criteria	S	U	NP	Comments
	Assessment				
1.	Assessed client understanding of need to collect urine from indwelling catheter				
2.	Assessed indwelling catheter for built—in port and type of material from which it is made				

Contd...

Contd...

Sl. No.	Performance Criteria	S	U	NP	Comments
	Nursing Diagnosis				
1.	Self care deficit urinary elimination				
	Planning				
1.	Uncontaminated urine specimen will be obtained from client catheter				
	Implementation				
1.	Washed hands				
2.	Clamped drainage tubing with clamp for 30 minutes				
3.	Informed client that the procedure to collect specimen from a catheter will begin				
4.	Wash hands and put on gloves				
5.	Position client so catheter is easily accessible				
6.	Cleansed entry port for needle with disinfectant swab				
7.	Insert needle at 30 degree angle just above where catheter is attached to drainage tube				
8.	Drawn urine into 20 mL syringe for routine urinalysis (3 mL for culture)				
9.	Transferred urine from syringe into lab specimen container				
10.	Placed tightly on container				
11.	Unclamped catheter and allow urine to flow into drainage bag				
12.	Disposed of soiled supplies, removed and discarded gloves and washed hands				
13.	Securely attached properly completed identification label and laboratory requisition to specimen				
14.	Sent specimen to laboratory immediately				
	Evaluation				
1.	Observed characteristics of urine and client discomfort				

Contd...

Contd...

Sl. No.	Performance Criteria	S	U	NP	Comments
	Recording and reporting				
1.	Recorded collection of specimen in nurses notes, time, date, appearance, color, odor of urine				
2.	Notified physician about laboratory result				

Signature of Student ---------------------------------------

Signature of Clinical Instructor --------------------------------

Performance Evaluation: Measuring Specific Gravity of Urine

Specific Gravity, the concentration of dissolved substances in water, can easily be measured by the nurse in any clinical setting. The most common mode is to place a urinometer with a mercury bulb in a cylinder containing urine. The density or concentration of urine determines the level at which the urinometer floats within the cylinder. If the urine is dilute, the urinometer tends to sink. Concentrated solutes in urine raise the level at which floats. This test requires only a few seconds to complete and can often provide useful information about the clients status of hydration and or kidney function and provide a parameter for the adjustment of fluid intake.

Procedure

Sl. No.	Performance Criteria	S	U	NP	Comments
	Assessment				
1.	Assessed client understanding of need to test specific gravity				
2.	Assessed client ability to collect specimen				
	Nursing diagnosis				
1.	• Fluid volume deficit • Fluid volume excess				
	Planning				
1.	Specific gravity will be accurately measured				
	Implementation				
1.	Explained procedure to client				
2.	Wash hands and put on clean, disposable gloves				

Contd...

Contd...

Sl. No.	Performance Criteria	S	U	NP	Comments
3.	Carefully poured fresh urine specimen into glass cylinder until it is 2/3 to 3/4 full				
4.	Placed urinometer in cylinder of urine and gently twirl top of stem				
5.	Waited until urinometer stops bobbing, then with urinometer scale at eye level, read point where urine level touches calibrated scale. Read scale at lowest point of meniscus for best accuracy				
6.	Discarded urine and washed cylinder and urinometer in cool water				
7.	Removed and discarded gloves and washed hands				
	Evaluation				
1.	Compared results with normal specific gravity				
	Recording and reporting				
1.	Recorded specific gravity reading and noted character of urine in nurses notes				
2.	Reported result to physician				

Signature of Student ---------------------------------------

Signature of Clinical Instructor ------------------------------

Performance Evaluation: Measuring Chemical Properties of Urine Glucose and Ketones

Sl. No.	Performance Criteria	S	U	NP	Comments
	Assessment				
1.	Assessed indication for urine test				
2.	Determined physician recommended specific type of reagent				
3.	Assessed client need to learn urine testing procedure				
	Nursing diagnosis				
1.	Ineffective management of urine testing				

Contd...

Contd...

Sl. No.	Performance Criteria	S	U	NP	Comments
	Planning				
	Developed individualized goals based on nursing diagnosis • Alterations in chemical properties of client urine will be detected • Client who requires daily or more frequent testing will be able to perform test independently				
	Implementation				
1.	Obtained double voided specimen				
2.	Asked client to collect random urine specimen and discard				
3.	Informed client to drink at least 8Z water or preferred liquid				
4.	30 to 40 minutes later, client collected another specimen				
5.	Performed glucose/ketone reagent test strip test				
6.	Immersed end of strip impregnated with chemical reagent into urine specimen				
7.	Removed strip immediately from specimen bottle and tap it gently against container side				
8.	Hold strip in horizontal position				
9.	Time for number of seconds specified on reagent strip container and compare color strip with chart				
10.	Disposed of reagent strip into trash				
11.	Used multistix reagent test strip to assess for glucose, ketones				
12.	Immersed end of chemical impregnated test strip into urine				
13.	Removed strip immediately from specimen container and taped it gently against container side				
14.	Hold strip in horizontal position				
15.	Time for number of seconds specified on test strip container and compare color of strip with color chart				

Contd...

Contd...

Sl. No.	Performance Criteria	S	U	NP	Comments
16.	Washed hands after removing and discarding gloves				
	Evaluation				
1.	Noted presence of glucose and ketones in the urine				
2.	Test result are positive for glucose				
	Recording and reporting				
1.	Recorded immediately in nurses glucose testing flow sheet				
2.	Reported to physician about the report				

Signature of Student ---------------------------------------

Signature of Clinical Instructor ------------------------------

Performance Evaluation: Measuring Blood Glucose Level after Skin Puncture

Sl. No.	Performance Criteria	S	U	NP	Comments
	Assessment				
1.	Assessed understanding of procedure and purpose				
2.	Determine if client knows how to performed test and the importance of glucose monitoring				
3.	Determined specific conditions required before sample collection with fasting after meals or after certain medications				
4.	Assessed area of skin to be used as puncture site-avoid areas of bruising, open lesions or abnormalities				
5.	Reviewed physician order				
6.	For client who performs test at home. Assessed ability to handle skin puncturing device				
	Nursing diagnosis				
1.	Altered health maintenance				

Contd...

Contd...

Sl. No.	Performance Criteria	S	U	NP	Comments
	Planning				
1.	**Develop individualized goals** • Client will experience minimal injury from skin puncture • Client will understand blood glucose testing				
	Expected outcomes • Client will be able to perform glucose monitoring using proper technique • Client will be able to monitor normal glucose level				
	Implementation				
1.	Washed hands before procedure				
2.	Instructed client to wash hands				
3.	Positioned client comfortably in chair or semi fowlers position in bed				
4.	Removed reagent strip from container and tightly sealed cap				
5.	Turned glucose meter on				
6.	Inserted strip in to glucose meter and make necessary adjustment (follow manufacturer's directions)				
7.	Applied disposable gloves				
8.	Selected puncture site				
9.	Hold finger to be punctured in dependent position while gently massaged finger to be punctured				
10.	Cleansed site with antiseptic swab and allowed to dry				
11.	Removed cover of lancet or blood letting device				
12.	Hold lancet perpendicular to puncture site and pierce finger or heel quickly in one continuous motion. Do not force lancet				
13.	Wiped away first droplet of blood with cotton ball (or as manufactures directions describe)				
14.	Squeezed puncture site until droplet formed				

Contd...

Contd...

Sl. No.	Performance Criteria	S	U	NP	Comments
15.	Hold reagent strip test pad close to drop of blood and Lightly transferred drop of blood to reagent strip test pad				
16.	Applied pressure to skin puncture site				
17.	Noted glucose reading on display				
18.	Turned meter off and disposed of test strip and cotton balls/swabs				
19.	Removed disposable gloves and disposed of properly				
20.	Washed hands				
21.	Shared test results with client				
	Evaluation				
1.	Compared present reading with normal levels				
2.	Inspected puncture site for bleeding or tissue injury				
3.	Enquired if client had any questions or concerns				
4.	Observed any unexpected outcomes				
	Recording and reporting				
1.	Recorded present readings in nurses notes, as well as action taken for abnormal readings				
2.	Administered insulin or hypoglycemic agents as prescribed				
3.	Provided diabetes diet as prescribed				
4.	Provided any explanations or teaching for client				
5.	Reported abnormal blood glucose levels to nurse incherage/physician				
6.	Record procedure and glucose level in nurses notes. Glycemic form diabetic chart				

Signature of Student --

Signature of Clinical Instructor ---------------------------------

CHAPTER

9

Performance Evaluation of Wound Care

Performance Evaluation: Assessment of Pressure Ulcer Development

Sl. No.	Performance Criteria	S	U	NP	Comments
	Assessment				
1.	Assessed the client upon admission such as • Client exposure to body fluid, urine, feces, wound drainage • Observed all pressure points, bony prominence • Observed underlying skin areas where tape, tubing, casts, splint contact with skin • Inspected the area of bony prominences-heels, ankles, knees, hips, sacral area, spinal area, shoulders and elbows • Observed perineal area for signs of redness, irritated skin • Determined potential and actual skin breakdown and noted				
	Nursing diagnosis				
1.	Impaired skin integrity related to pressure on bony prominence				
	Planning				
1.	Injury to client skin and underlying tissue will be reduced				
2.	Client ability to tolerate the position changes will improve				
	Implementation				
1.	Inspected condition of the skin regularly				
2.	Observed all devices for pressure point				
3.	Determined client ability to change and control body position				

Contd...

Contd...

Sl. No.	Performance Criteria	S	U	NP	Comments
4.	Evaluated frequently presence of friction and shear				
5.	Followed frequent change in position protocol				
6.	Provided pressure reducing support				
7.	Monitored toileting program, frequency of incontinence of urine and stool				
8.	Evaluated nutritional and laboratory values				
	Recording and reporting				
1.	Recorded client risk score				
2.	Recorded condition of skin under pressure in nurses notes				

Signature of Student --

Signature of Clinical Instructor --------------------------------

Performance Evaluation: Wound Management

Sl. No.	Performance Criteria	S	U	NP	Comments
	Assessment				
1.	Identified the phases of wound healing and states the difference between primary and secondary intention wound healing				
	Nursing diagnosis				
1.	Impaired skin integrity related to assessment data				
	Planning				
1.	Injury to client skin and underlying tissue will be reduced				
2.	States the purpose of various dressing materials				
	Implementation				
1.	Explained procedure to client				
2.	Assembled necessary equipment for wound care				

Contd...

Contd...

Sl. No.	Performance Criteria	S	U	NP	Comments
3.	Administered prescribed medication to the patient before changing dressing				
4.	Washed hands, applied gloves				
5.	Observed strict aseptic principles when performing the dressing change				
6.	Ensured that granulation tissue is kept moist and is not debrided				
7.	Ensured that exposed bones, tendons and muscles are kept moist with saline soaked gauze/oil emulsion gauze				
8.	Attempts to remove cellular debris and purulent exudates when cleaning the wound. Applied topical agents as prescribed • applied thin, even layer of ointment over necrotic areas of wound				
9.	Adhered to scheduled times for dressing change				
10.	Maintained sterility of wound drains				
11.	Changes dressing when they are soiled or saturated				
12.	Ensures that synthetic wound grafts are kept moist when dressing are applied				
13.	Protects skin from breakdown by using skin barrier				
14.	Obtained wound cultures as ordered				
15.	Removed gloves and dispose of soiled supplies, performed hand hygiene				
	Documentation				
1.	Documents all pertinent information in nurses notes				

Student Signature ----------------------

Supervisor Signature-------------------------

Performance Evaluation: Client With Surgical Drainage Tube

Sl. No.	Performance Criteria	S	U	NP	Comments
	Assessment				
1.	Identified types of surgical drain				
	Implementation				
1.	Decompress closed suction drain every 4 hours as needed				
2.	Changes drain dressing according to institutional policy				
3.	Ensures that drain bags are in a dependent position and that the tubing is not kinked				
4.	Ensures that sutures remain intact at the insertion site				
5.	Protects skin around drain site from breakdown by using skin barrier				
6.	Emetics collection chamber and measures drain output every 8 hours or as needed (exception, the collection chamber of the wall suction system may be emptied every 24 hours)				
7.	Assessed for an increased in output from abdominal drains during infusion of enteral feeding or medications, and notifies the physician as it occurs				
8.	When instilling continuous irrigation fluid through a drain, warms the fluid to body temperature and records the amount instilled				
9.	States rationale for care of specific drains				
	Recording and reporting				
1.	Documented all pertinent information				

Signature of Student ---------------------------------------

Signature of Clinical Instructor -------------------------------

Performance Evaluation: Management of Pressure Ulcers

Sl. No.	Performance Criteria	S	U	NP	Comments
	Assessment				
1.	Assessed client level of comfort				
	Nursing diagnosis				
1.	Impaired skin integrity related to pressure on bony prominence				
	Planning				
1.	Injury to client skin and underlying tissue will be reduced				
2.	Client ability to tolerate the position changes will improve				
	Implementation				
1.	Assembled needed supplies at bed side				
2.	Removed client linen to expose ulcer and surrounding skin				
3.	Gently washed skin surrounding ulcer with warm water				
4.	Cleansed ulcer thoroughly with normal saline				
5.	Applied topical agent as prescribed applied antiseptic agents correctly applied hydrogel agent correctly				
6.	Repositioned client comfortably				
	Recording and reporting				
1.	Recorded condition of skin under pressure in nurses notes				
2.	Recorded appearance of ulcer in nurses notes				
3.	Reported condition of ulcer to nurse in charge and physician				

Signature of Student ---------------------------------------

Signature of Clinical Instructor --------------------------------

Performance Evaluation: Applying an Abdominal Binder. T Binder or Breast Binder

Sl. No.	Performance Criteria	S	U	NP	Comments
	Assessment				
1.	Assessed signs and symptoms of impaired respirations				
2.	Observed level of skin integrity				
3.	Inspected for any surgical dressing				
4.	Identified client's comfort level				
5.	Gathered necessary data regarding size of binder based on assessment				
	Nursing diagnosis				
1.	Nursing diagnosis based on assessment data				
	Planning				
1.	Developed goals for client based on nursing diagnosis				
2.	Identified expected outcomes				
3.	Explained procedure to client				
	Implementation				
1.	Washed hands and applied gloves				
2.	Provided privacy				
3.	Positioned client in the supine position, head slightly elevated, knee slightly flexed				
4.	Assisted and asked client to roll to the side facing away from nurse. If there is an incision, instruct the client to support it with his or her hands				
5.	Placed fan-folded binder under the client with its upper border at the waist and lower border at the gluteal folds				
6.	Assisted the client to roll toward the nurse over the fan-folded binder				
7.	Reached over the client and straighten the fan-folded binder until it is smooth and wrinkle free				
8.	Placed binder ends under client				

Contd...

Contd...

Sl. No.	Performance Criteria	S	U	NP	Comments
9.	Instructed client to roll over ends				
10.	Smoothed ends on far side of bed				
11.	Assisted client to supine position				
12.	Adjusted binder				
13.	Closed binder correctly				
14.	Assessed adequacy of breathing and coughing				
15.	Assessed client comfort level				
16.	Adjusted binder as necessary				
	T- or Double T binders				
1.	Prepared for the application				
2.	Assisted the client to a dorsal recumbent position				
3.	Instructed client to raise hips				
4.	Checked the perineal rectal dressing				
5.	Placed the horizontal band (waistband) around the waist above the iliac crest				
6.	Brought the remaining strap (perineal strap) down the midback and through the perineal area to the lower abdomen				
7.	Attached the perineal strap to the waist band by overlapping them and securing with a horizontal safety pin				
8.	**Double T binder** Applied in the same manner but placed the perineal strap on either side of the genitalia				
9.	Instructed client regarding binder removal				
	Applying breast binder				
1.	Prepared for procedure				
2.	Helped the client to place her arms through the arm holes of the vest or placed the binder on bed with the strap open at top				
3.	Assisted client to a supine position on top of binder				

Contd...

Contd...

Sl. No.	Performance Criteria	S	U	NP	Comments
4.	Placed cotton padding under the breasts				
5.	Secured the binder safely at the nipple level with vertical safety pins or velcro closures				
6.	Continued securing below the center closure then above				
7.	Secured the last bottom closure with a horizontal safety pin				
8.	Monitored the client comfort and ability to breath adjust the binding as needed				
9.	Fastened straps with safety pin as required				
10.	Instructed client in self care				
	Evaluation				
1.	Observed skin integrity, comfort level ability to cough and deep breath				
	Recording and reporting				
1.	Reported ineffective lung expansion immediately to sister in charge/clinical instructor recorded necessary data in nurses' note.				

Signature of Student ---------------------------------------

Signature of Clinical Instructor ------------------------------

Performance Evaluation: Applying Elastic Bandage

Sl. No.	Performance Criteria	S	U	NP	Comments
	Assessment				
1.	Observed client's skin integrity				
2.	Observed cleanliness of dressing				
3.	Observed clients circulatory status				
4.	Reviewed clients medical record for physician order for application of elastic bandage				
5.	Identified client's knowledge level				

Contd...

Contd...

Sl. No.	Performance Criteria	S	U	NP	Comments
	Nursing diagnosis				
1.	Developed appropriate nursing diagnosis based on assessment data				
	Planning				
1.	Developed individualized goals for client based on nursing diagnosis				
2.	Identified expected outcomes				
3.	Explained procedure to client				
	Implementation				
1.	Washed hands and applied glove				
2.	Provided privacy				
3.	Assisted client to comfortable position. Held elastic bandage correctly				
4.	Applied bandage from distal point toward proximal boundary				
5.	Slightly stretched bandage as it was unrolled				
6.	Overlapped turns				
7.	Secured bandage				
8.	Washed hands				
	Evaluation				
1.	Checked circulation to the limb after application of bandage				
2.	Identified unexpected outcomes				
	Recording and reporting				
1.	Correctly documented treatment and clients response				

Signature of Student -------------------------------------

Signature of Clinical Instructor ------------------------------

Performance Evaluation: Assisting with the Application of Skin Traction

Sl. No.	Performance Criteria	S	U	NP	Comments
	Assessment				
1.	Determined the location of the injury, the purpose of the traction and which joints and muscles are immobilized				
2.	Examined the location for laceration, abrasions or achymosis				
3.	Assessed the neurovascular status of the affected area				
	Nursing diagnosis				
1.	Impaired physical mobility				
	Planning				
1.	Identified expected outcomes				
2.	Explained reasons for traction				
3.	Assessed clients' limbs applying traction for adequate circulatory and neuromuscular function				
	Implementation				
1.	Explained procedure to the client				
2.	Inspected the traction frame attached to the bed				
3.	Prepared client and area of the body to be placed in traction				
4.	Positioned the client as required				
5.	Placed specific traction equipment				
6.	Attached the bars, ropes and pulleys				
7.	Attached gently lowered traction weights				
8.	Assessed clients body alignment in traction				
9.	Elevated side rails				
10.	Returned unused materials to storage area				
11.	Washed hands				
12.	Inspected the traction frame attached to the bed to ensure that it will provide the correct amount and direction of force				

Contd...

Contd...

Sl. No.	Performance Criteria	S	U	NP	Comments
13.	Examined the knots in the ropes attached to the frame and weight carrier, to ensure safety				
	Evaluation				
1.	Reassessed the client for normal color, capillary refill, pulsations, movement, and sensation of the limbs for adequate circulation				
	Documentation				
1.	Recorded the type of traction, placed the amount of weight and physical response to traction				

Signature of Student ---------------------------------------

Signature of Clinical Instructor ------------------------------

CHAPTER

10

Performance Evaluation of Medication Administration

Performance Evaluation: Administering Oral Medication

Sl. No.	Performance Criteria	S	U	NP	Comments
	Assessment				
1.	Assessed for contraindications to client receiving oral medication, including difficulty in swallowing, nausea or vomiting, bowel inflammation or reduced peristalsis, recent gastrointestinal surgery, reduced peristalsis, reduced or absent bowel sounds, gastric suction, decreased level of consciousness				
2.	Checked client has no allergic to ordered drugs				
	Nursing diagnosis				
1.	Health seeking behavior				
	Planning				
1.	Prepared needed supplies and equipment				
2.	Identified expected outcomes				
3.	Compared medication administration record to physician order, adhered to principles of five rights of drug administration				
	Implementation				
1.	Checked physician written order. check client name, and drug name, dosage, route of administration and time for administration				
2.	Identified client by comparing name on card form or ask client to state full name				

Contd...

Contd...

Sl. No.	Performance Criteria	S	U	NP	Comments
3.	Determined the dosage ordered is within usual dosage range				
4.	Removed tablet from bottle, by pouring required numbers into medication cup without touching the drug				
5.	Gently poured drug one by one into mouth, without rush				
6.	Administered drug properly				
	Evaluation				
1.	Observed for significant changes and also informed client to report any discomfort				
	Documentation				
1.	Recorded drug admistered to client in nurses' progress notes				

Signature of Student --

Signature of Clinical Instructor ------------------------------

Performance Evaluation: Administering Subcutaneous, Intradermal and Intramuscular Injection

Sl. No.	Performance Criteria	S	U	NP	Comments
	Assessment				
1.	Assessed indications for proper route for medication				
2.	Assess medical history of allergies				
3.	Washed hands				
4.	Prepared needed equipment and supplies				
5.	Assessed site last injection, intended injection site				
6.	Determined appropriate size and gauze of needle				

Contd...

Contd...

Sl. No.	Performance Criteria	S	U	NP	Comments
	Nursing diagnosis				
1.	Altered comfort, anxiety related to pain from injection				
	Planning				
1.	• State the purpose of injection • Client will verbalize minimum discomfort related to injection				
	Implementation				
1.	• Explained procedure to client • Washed hands				
2.	Prepared medication, adhering to the five rights of drug administration				
3.	Identified client by reading identification label or call the name				
4.	Selected injection site appropriate site for client size and age **Sub-Q**—palpate site for masses, by grasping skin fold at site with thumb and forefinger **IM**—note integrity and size of muscle and palpated for tenderness **ID**—noted lesions, any discoloration of forearm, select site three to four finger width below anticubital space and hand width above wrist				
5.	Assist client into position for comfort and easy visibility of injection site				
6.	Kept sheet/gown draped over body parts not requiring exposure				
7.	Instructed client lie flat on side or prone or have client sit, depending on site chosen				
8.	Cleansed site with antiseptic swab				
9.	Removed cap from needle by pulling it straight off				
10.	Holding syringe correctly between thumb and fore finger of dominant hand				

Contd...

Contd...

Sl. No.	Performance Criteria	S	U	NP	Comments
11.	**Intra muscular injection** Positioned nondominant hand at proper anatomical land mark and spread skin tightly. Inject needle quickly at 90 degree angle into muscle				
12.	Aspirated drug if drug appear in syringe remove needle discard medication and syringe, and repeat procedure				
13.	Injected medication slowly				
14.	Withdrawn needle while applying alcohol swab gently above or over injection site				
15.	Massaged skin lightly				
16.	**Intradermal** With nondominant hand, stretched skin over site with forefinger. With needle almost against client skin insert it slowly with bevel up at a 5 to 15 degree angle until resistance is felt. Then advanced needle through epidermis to approximately 3 mm below skin surface. Needle tip can be seen through skin				
17.	Injected medication, slowly. Normally resistance is felt				
18.	While injecting medication, noticed that small bleb approximately 6 mm appeared in skin surface				
19.	Withdrawn needle while applying alcohol swab				
20.	Applied gentle pressure. Not massaged				
21.	Assisted client to comfortable position				
22.	**Subcutaneous** Spread skin tightly across injection site with nondominant hand				

Contd...

Contd...

Sl. No.	Performance Criteria	S	U	NP	Comments
23.	Injected needle quickly and firmly at 45 to 9o degree angle below tissue fold				
24.	Injected medication slowly				
25.	Discarded an uncapped needle or needle enclosed in safety shield and attached syringe in appropriately labeled container				
26.	Washed hands				
	Evaluation				
1.	Returned to room and ask if client feels acute pain burning, numbness or tingling at injection site. Observe for allergic reaction after injection				
2.	Returned to evaluate response to medication in 10 to 30 min				
3.	For ID injection, drawn circle around perimeter of injection site with pen				
	Recording and reporting				
1.	Recorded drug administered time, dosage, route and observation in nurses notes For ID injection recorded area of injection, amount and type of testing substance, and date and time on medication record				
2.	Reported abnormalities to physician immediately				

Signature of Student -------------------------------------

Signature of Clinical Instructor ------------------------------

Performance Evaluation: Mixing Medication from Two Vials

Occasionally, the nurse must mix medications from two vials or from a vial and an ample. Mixing medications from a vial and ample is simple, by adding air to the ampoule then withdraw the medication. The nurse first prepares medications from the vial first and then, using the same syringe and needle withdraws medication from the ampule.

Sl. No.	Performance Criteria	S	U	NP	Comments
	Assessment				
1.	Verified the physician medication order				
2.	Determined medications to be mixed and sterility of vials/ ampoules. Determined correct dose and amount				
	Implementation				
1.	Assembled supplies at clean working area at treatment room				
2.	Wash and dried hands				
3.	Taken syringe and aspirate volume of air equipment to first medications dosage (vial A)				
4.	Stand vial A upright –insert needle. inject air into vial A, making sure needle does not touch solution				
5.	Withdrawn needle and syringe and then aspirate air equivalent to second medication dose (vial B)				
6.	Stand vial B upright insert needle into vial B, inject air, invert vial then fill syringe with prescribed volume of medication from vial B				
7.	Withdrawn needle and syringe from vial by pulling on barrel. Checked the dose				
8.	Determined, at which point on the syringe scale, the combined volume of medication measures				
9.	Inserted needle into a vial A, being careful not to push plunger and expel medication into vial, invert vial and carefully withdraw desired amount of medication into syringe				
10.	Withdrawn needle and expelled excess air from syringe				
11.	Changed needle on syringe. Do not remove cap or sheath from needle				

Contd...

Contd...

Sl. No.	Performance Criteria	S	U	NP	Comments
12.	Disposed off soiled needle and supplies in proper receptacles				
13.	Wash and dry hands				

Signature of Student --------------------------------------

Signature of Clinical Instructor -------------------------------

Performance Evaluation: Teaching Client How to Administer Self Insulin Injections

Sl. No.	Performance Criteria	S	U	NP	Comments
	Assessment				
1.	Assessed client readiness to learn				
2.	Assessed level of client understanding of procedure				
3.	Assessed clients ability to hold and manipulate a syringe and vial				
4.	Assessed client visual ability by having read numbers on insulin syringe or directions on vial of insulin				
5.	Assessed clients understanding of diabetes and purpose and action and reason why insulin is required				
6.	Assessed family member's interest and ability to provide injections				
7.	Assessed drug dose and schedule client is ordered to receive at home				
8.	Assessed clients existing knowledge regarding technique for self injection				
	Nursing diagnosis				
1.	Health seeking behavior regarding self administration of insulin				
	Planning				
1.	Assessed individualized objectives for teaching plan				

Contd...

Contd...

Sl. No.	Performance Criteria	S	U	NP	Comments
2.	Identified expected outcomes • Correctly manipulate parts of syringe and needle without contaminating them • Correctly prepare ordered dose in insulin syringe describes purpose for rotating sites				
3.	Provided adequate time for teaching session				
	Implementation				
1.	Have client wash hands. Explained importance of hand washing				
2.	Allowed client opportunity to manipulate syringe parts. Explain which parts must remain sterile and which can be touched				
3.	Asked client to compare syringe unit scale with label on insulin vial				
4.	Discussed clients to know the prescribed dosage				
5.	Demonstrated technique for mixing insulin in vial by gently rolling bottle between hands. Then allow client to mix the vial, never shake vial				
6.	Shown steps to prepare insulin in syringe and used simple terms during explanations • Wipe off top of vial with alcohol swab and remove needle cover • Pull plunger out to same number of units to be removed from vial. This pulls air into syringe • Push needle slowly into rubber on top of vial while holding syringe barrel carefully. Do not blend needle • Push in plunger to push in air into bottle this prevent vacuum • Hold vial and syringe together turn both upside down • Slowly pull back on plunger to number of units of insulin to be given				

Contd...

Contd...

Sl. No.	Performance Criteria	S	U	NP	Comments
	• Check for clear air bubbles inside syringe • Remove syringe from vial by pulling it straight out, pull back slightly on plunger and then push it back to correct number of units				
7.	Pointed out proper injection sites on client body				
8.	Explained importance of rotating injection site				
9.	Asked client to select injection site				
10.	Explained steps while administering injections, in his own understanding				
11.	Encouraged questions for client				
12.	Washed hands				
	Evaluation				
1.	Have client prepare syringe using saline or sterile water instead of insulin				
2.	Have client explain usual insulin dose and type				
3.	Asked client to prepare injection site and explain importance of rotating sites				
4.	Identified unexpected outcomes				
	Recording and reporting				
1.	Described in nurses notes content or skills taught to client and client's ability to perform skill				
2.	Follow up activities				
3.	Explained, client may need to practice several different steps of the procedure with assistance before performing each skill independently				

Signature of Student --------------------------------------

Signature of Clinical Instructor ------------------------------

Performance Evaluation: Administering Skin Applications (Topical Administration)

Sl. No.	Performance Criteria	S	U	NP	Comments
	Assessment				
1.	Referred physician drug order				
2.	Referred pertinent drug information				
3.	Determined the specific location of the application				
4.	Checked client history of allergies in general and skin reaction in specific				
5.	Assessed amount of topical agent required and direction for use				
6.	Verified clients knowledge regarding medication therapy				
7.	Observed if the client is awake, alert and able to cooperate for a sublingual or buccal medication				
8.	Assessed client ability to self administer medication				
	Nursing diagnosis				
1.	• Impaired skin integrity potential or actual • Health seeking behaviors related to knowledge deficit				
	Planning				
1.	The client will be without an allergic or inflammatory response to the topically applied medication				
	Implementation				
1.	Prepared to administer the medication, explain procedure to the client				
2.	Washed hands, arranged supplies at bed side, and applied gloves				
3.	Closed door or curtain for privacy and positioned client comfortably				
4.	Lowered the top bed covers and expose the designated area of the client skin inspect the skin integrity				

Contd...

Contd...

Sl. No.	Performance Criteria	S	U	NP	Comments
5.	Washed affected area of skin before application				
6.	Allowed skin to air dry or patted lightly to dry				
7.	Put on gloves Applied topical agent while skin still damp				
8.	Used correct procedure when applying any of following cream ointment or oil based lotion, antianginal ointment, patch, aerosol spray, suspension based lotion powder				
9.	Covered skin area with dressing when ordered				
10.	Assured client in returning to comfortable position after application				
11.	Removed gloves, properly disposed of soiled supplies and washed hands after procedure				
	Evaluation				
1.	Evaluated significant others knowledge of prescribed medication				
2.	Observed client administering medication				
3.	Assessed condition of skin between applications				
4.	Identified any side effect				
	Recording and reporting				
1.	Recorded in nurses notes condition of skin before applying topical agent				
2.	Recorded application of topical agent				
3.	Reported any abnormalities of skin condition to nurse in charge or physician				

Signature of Student ---------------------------------------

Signature of Clinical Instructor ------------------------------

Performance Evaluation: Starting Intravenous Infusion

Sl. No.	Performance Criteria	S	U	NP	Comments
	Assessment				
1.	Reviewed physician fluid replacement order				
2.	Assessed the indication for IV therapy				
3.	Identified client and explained procedure				
	Nursing diagnosis				
1.	Developed appropriate nursing diagnosis based on assessment data				
	Planning				
1.	Developed individualized objectives plan - verifies the components and additives with the physician prescription before administration				
	Implementation				
1.	Prepared solution and tubing, maintained aseptic technique when opening sterile packages and IV solution. Clamp tubing uncap spike				
2.	Inserted infusion set in to entry site on bag/bottle as manufacturer directs				
3.	Removed cap at end of tubing released clamp and allow fluid to flow until all bubble have flown out disappeared. Close clamp and recap end of tubing				
4.	Selected an appropriate site and palpated accessible veins				
5.	Assembled IV fluids and equipment				
6.	Applied tourniquet 10 to 12 cm (4–5 inch) above insertion site				
7.	Cleansed the entry site with firm, concentric circular motion outward from insertion site using povidone iodine solution and allowed to dry				

Contd...

Contd...

Sl. No.	Performance Criteria	S	U	NP	Comments
8.	Hold the needle bevel up and inserted it at 20 to 30° angle with smooth motion and entered				
9.	Quickly removed protective cap of IV tubing and attached it to the cannula				
10.	Started the flow of solution promptly by releasing the clamp on the tube				
11.	Looped the tubing near the site entry and anchored with tape				
12.	Adjusted the rate of solution flow according to amount prescribed				
13.	Marked the date, time and type and size of the cannula used for the infusion on the tape anchoring the tubing				
14.	Removed all equipment and disposed in proper manner, washed hands				
	Evaluation				
1.	Inspects the IV catheter site with the dressing change for evidence of infection and infiltration				
2.	Consults appropriate sources for the necessary information regarding unfamiliar medications				
3.	Follows hospital guidelines for changing IV tubing, fluid bags and dressing and rotating catheter sites				
	Recording and reporting				
1.	Recorded the procedure and client response, time site device used and solution and informed to sister in charge				
2.	Returned to check flow rate and observed for infiltration frequently				

Signature of Student -------------------------------------

Signature of Clinical Instructor ------------------------------

Performance Evaluation: Client with a Continuous Medication Infusion

Sl. No.	Performance Criteria	S	U	NP	Comments
	Assessment				
1.	Identifies the mode of action, indications, contraindications, and adverse reactions of the medication infusion				
2.	Calculates the proper concentration and rate of infusion, states the therapeutic range of the medication infusion, and documents the dose hourly				
	Implementation				
1.	Administers the medications via volumetric infusion pump				
2.	Monitors the client hemodynamic response continuously as per the protocols				
3.	Tirates the medication infusion to obtain the desired results				
4.	Determines compatibility of medications before administering concurrently through the same IV access				
5.	Monitors the serum concentration of certain medication infusion to prevent toxicity				
	Recording and reporting				
1.	Recorded the medication infusion time started, drop factors, expected time to complete				
2.	Reported to physician any adverse effect and time of infusion started				

Signature of Student --------------------------------------

Signature of Clinical Instructor ------------------------------

Performance Evaluation: Client with Transfusion of Blood and Blood Products

Transfusion of blood and blood products is a very common medical procedures in the practice of modern medicine. Nursing staff plays a very important and crucial role in the transfusion procedure, as they are called upon to procure blood and blood products from the blood transfusion laboratory and conduct and supervise the transfusion

Sl. No.	Performance Criteria	S	U	NP	Comments
	Assessment				
1.	Determined client knows reasons for transfusion				
2.	Verified client has had a transfusion or transfusion reaction in the past				
3.	Explained procedure to the client, obtained consent for transfusion				
	Implementation				
1.	Verified physician order				
2.	Washed hands and dried				
3.	Obtained blood products from blood bank according to agency policy				
4.	Verified blood for room temperature				
5.	Verified blood screening test done				
6.	Hanged container of 0.9% normal saline with blood administration set to initiate IV infusion and follow administration of blood				
7.	Started intravenous with no 18 catheter				
8.	Completed identification and checked as required by agency policy				
9.	Verified identification and checks donor and recipient, name blood groups and type				
10.	Verified that ABO groups and Rh type are the same and expiration date				
	Inspected blood for clots				
11.	Taken baseline set of vital signs prior to beginning transfusion				

Contd...

Contd...

Sl. No.	Performance Criteria	S	U	NP	Comments
12.	Started infusion of the blood product in line filter with blood				
13.	Started administration slowly				
14.	Observed client for flushing dyspnea, itching, hives or rash or any transfusion reaction				
15.	Maintain the prescribed flow rate and assess frequently for transfusion reaction. Stop				
16.	When transfusion completed started 0.9% normal saline				
	Recording and reporting				
1.	Recorded administration of blood, time started group and type				
2.	Reported to physician blood transfusion completed and no reaction noted				
3.	Returned bag to blood bank according to agency policy				

Signature of Student ---------------------------------------

Signature of Clinical Instructor -------------------------------

Performance Evaluation: Assisting Intravenous Cut Down

Cut down or venous section is a small incision to insert a cannula or catheter directly into the vein or artery specially using lower extremities. During emergency period or when vein is not accessible for infusion especially like burns cases.

Sl. No.	Performance Criteria	S	U	NP	Comments
	Assessment				
1.	Ensure surgeon or physician wanted to perform cut down				
2.	Obtained consent by client or relatives				
3.	Positioned client to enable full exposure of the site				

Contd...

Contd...

Sl. No.	Performance Criteria	S	U	NP	Comments
4.	Arranged cut down set from CSSD, (Kept ready dressing materials and Set by bed side)				
	Implementation				
1.	Prepared IV fluids and kept ready as per instruction				
2.	Assisted surgeon to perform cut down by supplying needed materials				
3.	Opened and poured betadine directly from container to gallipots				
4.	The surgeon cleans the skin, drape sterile towels and proceeds with procedure				
5.	Assisted surgeon for suturing the site and dressing				
6.	Connected IV fluids to the IV cut down site				
7.	Position the client on comfortable position				
8.	Removed all equipment and disposed in proper manner, washed hands				
	Recording and reporting				
1.	Recorded time and site of cut down				
2.	Recorded type of IV fluids started				
3.	Reported to charge nurse about the procedure				

Signature of Student --------------------------------------

Signature of Clinical Instructor ------------------------------

Performance Evaluation: Ear Irrigation

Irrigation of the external auditory canal to remove discharges from the canal, to facilitate removal of cerumen or foreign bodies and to apply heat to the tissues of the ear canal.

Nursing alert: Ask the client if he has a history of draining ears or if he had a perforation or other complications from previous ear irrigation. If the reply is affirmative, check with the physician before proceeding with the irrigation.

Sl. No.	Performance Criteria	S	U	NP	Comments
	Assessment				
1.	Used cotton applicator to remove discharge on outer ear				
2.	Placed kidney basin close to the client head and under the ear				
3.	Temperature of the solution tested by allowing some to run on inner aspect of wrist should be 35 to 40.6 degree centigrade				
	Implementation				
1.	Gently pulled the outer ear upward and backward				
2.	Placed tip of syringe at the opening of the ear and gently stream of the fluid against the sides of canal				
3.	Observed for sign of pain and dizziness				
4.	Irrigated ear to dislodge the wax				
5.	Positioned a piece of cotton wool at the entrance of the canal				
6.	Dispose of the equipment				
7.	Wash and dry hands				
	Recording and reporting				
1.	Recorded procedure in nurses notes				
2.	Reported to physician the result of procedure				

Signature of Student --

Signature of Clinical Instructor --------------------------------

Performance Evaluation: Instillation of Ear Drops

Instillation of ear drops, involves dropping, a prescribed solution into the external auditory canal from a dropper.

Sl. No.	Performance Criteria	S	U	NP	Comments
	Assessment				
1.	Explained procedure to the client				
2.	Collected and prepared equipment				
	Implementation				
1.	Assisted the client to sit in an upright position with his head tilted slightly from the affected ear				
2.	Checked the drug prescription with the ear drops label and expiry date				
3.	Washed and dried hands				
4.	Pulled the pinna of the ear gently in an upward and backward direction				
5.	Insert the prescribed number of ear drops into the canal				
6.	Position a piece of cotton wool at the entrance of the canal				
7.	Disposed of the equipment				
8.	Washed hands				
	Recording and reporting				
1.	Recorded procedure in nurses notes				
2.	Reported to physician the result of procedure				

Signature of Student --

Signature of Clinical Instructor ------------------------------

CHAPTER

11

Performance Evaluation of Higher Nursing Procedures

Performance Evaluation: Oxygen Therapy–Cannula Method

Sl. No.	Performance Criteria	S	U	NP	Comments
	Assessment				
1.	Assessed client need for oxygen				
2.	Verified physician order				
3.	Explained procedure to the patient				
4.	Observed clients airway and removed secretion if any				
	Nursing diagnosis				
1.	Impaired gas exchange				
	Planning				
1.	Placed no smoking sign on the client side, explain dangers of smoking when oxygen is on flow				
2.	Identified expected outcomes • Patient will be free from hypoxia • Patient will be able to breath normally				
	Implementation				
1.	Washed hands, set up oxygen equipment and humidifier				
2.	Attached humidifier to base flow meter				
3.	Attached oxygen tubing and nasal cannula to humidified oxygen or gas source				
4.	Placed tip of cannula to patient nares and adjust straps around ear for snug fit, fixed the elastic band behind head or under chin				
5.	Adjusted oxygen flow rate to prescribed dosage and verified that water in humidifier was bubbling				
6.	Assessed humidity source every 4 hours and changed container every 24 hours				
7.	Observed for gagging, vomiting when necessary				

Contd...

Contd...

Sl. No.	Performance Criteria	S	U	NP	Comments
	Evaluation				
1.	Reassessed client to determine response to administration of oxygen by nasal cannula				
2.	Observed the client's nose and ears for skin breakdown				
	Recording				
1.	Recorded in nurses progress notes, starting time, flow rate and response of the client				

Signature of Student --

Signature of Clinical Instructor -------------------------------

Performance Evaluation: Obtaining Arterial Blood Gas Sample

Sl. No.	Performance Criteria	S	U	NP	Comments
	Assessment				
1..	Identified the indication for obtaining arterial blood samples				
	Implementation				
1.	Performed Allen test				
2.	Obtained the arterial blood sample				
3.	Placed the heparinized syringe with the arterial blood sample in a small container of ice				
4.	Informed the laboratory personnel of the client temperature to allow temperature correction of the blood sample				
	Evaluation				
1.	Compared the normal range of ABGS result to client result				
	Recording and reporting				
1.	Recorded ABGS result in nurses notes				
2.	Reported laboratory findings to physician				

Signature of Student --

Signature of Clinical Instructor -------------------------------

Performance Evaluation: Chest Drainage Tube Maintenance (Water Seal)

Sl. No.	Performance Criteria	S	U	NP	Comments
	Assessment				
1.	Assessed type of drainage system				
2.	Assessed base line data, breath sound, respiratory rate, pulse rate, temperature, blood gases etc.				
	Nursing diagnosis				
1.	Ineffective breathing pattern related to decreased lung expansion				
	Planning				
1.	Client will show nonlabored respiration and respiratory rate within normal limit				
	Implementation				
1.	Washed hands and organized equipments				
2.	Unwraped drainage system and placed it up right				
3.	Filled bottle or chambers to appropriate level				
4.	**One bottle system** • Placed funnel in port or tubing leading to long rod and fill bottle with solution until end of rod is 2 cm below fluid level **Two or three bottle chamber system** • Poured fluid into suction control port until designated amount is reached indicating the 20 cm water pressure level • The suction control bottle in a two bottle system is the bottle with the long rod. The closed chamber drainage system is more commonly used				
5.	Connected tubing from client to tubing entering drainage collection bottle or chamber				
6.	When changing drainage system, asked client to take deep breath, hold it and bear down slightly while tubing is being changed quickly				
7.	Adjusted suction flow regulator until quiet bubbling is noted in suction control chamber				
	Evaluation				
1.	Observed water seal drainage chamber for bubbling, (suspect air leak if bubbling is present) checked security of tube				
2.	Marked drainage in collection chamber/bottle				

Contd...

Contd...

Sl. No.	Performance Criteria	S	U	NP	Comments
3.	If drainage slows or stops consulted the physician				
4.	Milking • Grasped tube close to chest and squeezed tube between fingers and palm of hand • Observed drainage system below level of client chest				
5.	Checked for fluctuation in water seal chamber with respirations				
	Recording				
1.	Reported to nurse incharge significant changes during monitoring				

Signature of Student ---------------------------------------

Signature of Clinical Instructor ------------------------------

Performance Evaluation: Endotracheal Tube Suctioning-Endotracheal Tube Maintenance

Sl. No.	Performance Criteria	S	U	NP	Comments
	Assessment				
1.	Assessed airway patency (clear inspiratory and expiratory breath sounds)				
2.	Assessed endotracheal tube stability, securely placed tubing and properly inflated cuff				
3.	Assessed apparatus settings and oxygen level				
	Nursing diagnosis				
1.	• Ineffective airway clearance related to weak cough • Anxiety related to inability to breath effectively				
	Planning				
1.	• Client will be able to maintain a patent airway • Demonstrate adequate oxygenation • Care giver will maintain oxygenation during procedure				
	Implementation				
1.	Explained procedure to the patient and washed hands				
2.	Determined length of catheter to be inserted, measured distance from tip of nose to earlobe				
3.	Applied gloves				

Contd...

Contd...

Sl. No.	Performance Criteria	S	U	NP	Comments
4.	Positioned client on side or back with head or bed elevated				
5.	Turned suction machine and placed finger over end of tubing				
6.	Opened sterile irrigation solution and poured into sterile cup				
7.	Placed towel under client chin				
8.	Set oxygen on ambu breathing bag and turn on full flow				
9.	Delivered ventilation, administered three to five deep ventilation or allowed client to take three to five deep breath if client is able to do				
10.	Performed suction maneuvers, continued insertion until resistance is met or coughing is stimulated. (Suction should not be applied more than 10 to 12 seconds)				
11.	Placed tip of suction catheter in sterile solution and applied suction for 1 to 2 seconds				
12.	Deflated ET tube cuff and repeated suctioning				
13.	Re inflated cuff to appropriate pressure				
14.	Suctioned oral airway and performed oral care				
15.	Disconnected suction catheter from suction tubing turned off suction machine				
16.	Positioned client with head of bed at 45° and side rail up				
17.	Properly disposed or stored supplies/equipment				
	Recording				
1.	Recorded suctioning in nursing progress notes Informed nurse incharge any significant response of the client				

Signature of Student ---------------------------------------

Signature of Clinical Instructor --------------------------------

Performance Evaluation: Postural Drainage

Sl. No.	Performance Criteria	S	U	NP	Comments
	Assessment				
1.	Assessed respiration and breath sounds are clear				
	Nursing Diagnosis				
1.	Ineffective airway clearance related to excessive secretions				
	Planning				
1.	Client will maintain clear air way within normal limit				
	Implementation				
1.	Explained and demonstrated procedure to client				
2.	Washed hands and organized equipment				
3.	Administered bronchodilators, expectorants or warm liquids as per ordered				
4.	Encouraged the client to void				
5.	Positioned client • Sitting upright in bed (or chair) performed therapy to right and left chest (to drain anterior right and left apical segment) • Leaning forward in sitting position performed therapy to back (to drain right and left segment) • Lying flat on back performed therapy to right and left chest (to drain anterior segment) • Lying on abdomen, tilted to right or left side performed therapy to right or left back (to drain posterior segments)				
6.	Maintained client in position until chest percussion and vibration are completed (approximately 5 minutes) to loosen secretion in target area				
7.	Assisted client into position for coughing or for suctioning of trachea				
8.	Positioned client to drain next target area and repeated percussion and vibration				
9.	Repeated percussion, vibration, and cough/suction sequence until identified lung fields have been drained				
10.	Assessed breath sounds in targeted lung fields				
11.	Assisted client with mouth care				
12.	Positioned client in bed with head of bed elevated 45° (or more)				

Contd...

Contd...

Sl. No.	Performance Criteria	S	U	NP	Comments
13.	Turned client to side with pillow at back				
	Recording and reporting				
1.	Recorded procedure in nurses progress notes				
2.	Reported to clinical instructor and nurse in charge about response of the patient for the procedure				

Signature of Student ---

Signature of Clinical Instructor --------------------------------

Performance Evaluation Tracheotomy Suctioning

Sl. No.	Performance Criteria	S	U	NP	Comments
	Assessment				
1.	Assessed type of tracheotomy tube, respiratory status and secretions				
	Nursing diagnosis				
1.	• Ineffective airway clearance related to weak cough • Anxiety related to inability to breath effectively				
	Planning				
1.	• Attain and maintain a patent airway, as indicated by respiratory rate of 14 to 20 breaths per minute • Client will maintain respiration without cyanosis				
	Implementation				
1.	Explained procedure to the patient and washed hands				
2.	Applied gloves				
3.	Positioned client on side/ back with head of bed elevated				
4.	Turned suction machine and placed finger over end of tubing attached to suction machine				
5.	Opened sterile irrigation solution and poured into sterile cup				
6.	Placed towel or drape on client chest under tracheotomy				
7.	Asked client to take several deep breaths with tracheotomy collar intact				
8.	Removed tracheotomy collar or ambu bag				

Contd...

Contd...

Sl. No.	Performance Criteria	S	U	NP	Comments
9.	Inserted catheter approximately 6 inches into inner cannula (or until resistance is met or cough reflex is stimulated) by making sure finger is not covering the opening of suction port				
10.	Encouraged client to cough				
11.	Withdrawn catheter in a circular motion, rotating catheter between thumb and finger (Intermittent release and application of suction during withdrawal is recommended. Is recommended). Applied suction for no more than 10 to 15 seconds				
12.	Placed tip of suction catheter in sterile solution and applied suction for 1 to 2 seconds				
13.	Allowed client to take about five breath while auscultating bronchial breath sounds				
14.	Repeated step 9-13 once or twice if secretion are still present				
15.	Positioned client for comfort				
16.	Washed hands				
	Recording				
1.	• Recorded suctioning in nursing progress notes • Informed sister incharge any significant response of the client				

Signature of Student ---------------------------------------

Signature of Clinical Instructor --------------------------------

Performance Evaluation: Measuring Central Venous Pressure

Central venous pressure (CVP) is a measure of the pressure within the right atrium of the heart. CVP can be measured using a manometer attached to the intravenous fluid line, in terms of fluid pressure in column of the manometer.

Sl. No.	Performance Criteria	S	U	NP	Comments
	Assessment				
1.	Identified client required central venous pressure monitoring				
2.	Informed procedure to the client				
3.	Checked articles required for CVP measurement				

Contd...

Contd...

Sl. No.	Performance Criteria	S	U	NP	Comments
	Implementation				
1.	Wash hands				
2.	Positioned client in supine position with no pillows under head				
3.	Verified manometer on an IV pole, it is zeroed at X mark				
4.	Verified and connect IV fluid, and 3 way stopcock and flush the other two ports				
5.	Connected the CVP manometer to the upper port of the stopcock				
6.	Connected the CVP tubing from the client to the second side port of the stopcock				
7.	Turned stopcock off to client and fill manometer with IV fluids to the 20 cm mark above the anticipated reading				
8.	Hold manometer at the phlebostatic axis and turn the stopcock off to the IV fluid				
9.	Watch as the fluid falls in the manometer take the central venous pressure reading when fluids stabilizes				
10.	Turned the stopcock off to the manometer				
11.	Reposition the client				
12.	Kept the manometer in an upright position (usually hanging from IV pole)				
13.	Wash and dry hands				
	Recording and reporting				
1.	Recorded CVP pressure reading in nurses notes				
2.	Reported to physician about significant readings				

Signature of Student ---------------------------------------

Signature of Clinical Instructor ------------------------------

Performance Evaluation: Assisting with Arterial Puncture

Arterial pressure is the stress exerted by the circulating blood on the walls of the arteries. The amount of arterial pressure in an individual is the product of the cardiac output and the systemic vascular resistance.

Procedure: Assisting for collection of blood sample from an artery by performing an arterial puncture.

Sl. No.	Performance Criteria	S	U	NP	Comments
	Assessment				
1.	Identified client required arterial puncture				
2.	Assembled necessary equipment for insertion of an arterial catheter				
3.	Assessed client vital signs				
4.	Assessed client oxygen saturation level				
	Implementation				
1.	Perform Allen test (radial artery is selected)				
2.	Filled 2 mL syringe with heparine, expelled excess air				
3.	Wash hands and don gloves				
4.	Placed pad under forearm				
5.	Assessed radial artery pulsation				
6.	Placed needle at 45–60 degree angle advanced into the artery. Once felt needle in position blood will fill the syringe				
7.	After blood is obtained withdraw needle and applied firm pressure over the puncture site with dry gauze for 5 to 10 minutes and applied firm pressure dressing				
8.	Send labeled, iced specimen to the laboratory immediately with lab requisition				
	Evaluation				
1.	Palpated the pulse distal to the puncture site, observed puncture site for temperature, numbness				
	Recording				
1.	Recorded procedure in nurses note and who performed the procedure				
2.	Wash and dry hands				

Signature of Student --------------------------------------

Signature of Clinical Instructor ------------------------------

Performance Evaluation: Arterial Pressure Monitoring

Procedure

Sl. No.	Performance Criteria	S	U	NP	Comments
	Assessment				
1.	Identified client required arterial pressure monitoring				
2.	Performed Allen test				
3.	Assessed client vital signs				
4.	Assessed client oxygen saturation level				
	Implementation				
1.	Placed the air filled interface of the transducer system at the level of the cannulated artery				
2.	Balanced /zeros the transducer to atmospheric pressure every 4 hours				
3.	Identifies the normal arterial wave form and troubleshoots deviation as necessary				
4.	Compared the direct arterial pressure measurement with the indirect sphygmomanometer measurements				
5.	Assessed pulse, color, sensation and temperature distal to the insertion site every 2 to 4 hours				
6.	Observed the skin at the site				
7.	Changed the flush solution, tubing and dressing				
8.	Drawn blood samples from the arterial catheter using the proximal stopcock				
	Record and reporting				
1.	Recorded arterial pressure in nurses notes				
2.	Informed to physician the significant pressure				

Signature of Student --

Signature of Clinical Instructor --------------------------------

Performance Evaluation: Assisting Endotracheal Intubation

Endotracheal tube is inserted into the trachea via the mouth or nose, in addition connecting for ventilators the ET tube a long slender, hollow tube provides as table airway and facilitates removal of secretions. The ET tube also prevents verbal communication. It passes through the vocal cords. Oral intubation is usually used for short-term airway management.

Sl. No.	Performance Criteria	S	U	NP	Comments
	Assessment				
1.	Identified indication for ET intubation				
2.	Explained procedure to the client/relatives				
3.	Obtained client /relatives consent				
4.	Assessed risk factors for intubation				
5.	Arranged required articles				
	Implementation				
1.	Placed client in supine position with head is hyper extended				
2.	Loose teeth are removed, the lower aspect of the neck is flexed and mouth is opened				
3.	Used oxygen mask to provide oxygen through mouth				
4.	Handed over laryngoscope, and suction to doctor				
5.	Provided lubricated endotracheal tube				
6.	Assisted while endotracheal tube is introduced into the trachea and removed stiletto				
7.	Immediately after ET tube insertion, tube placement is verified by auscultation and chest X-ray.				
8.	Assessed oxygen saturation level for ET tube placement				
9.	Connected ambu bag with oxygen attached to the endotracheal tube and continued bagging				
10.	Inflated cuff of the endotracheal tube with 10 mL of air				
11.	Noted point at which the tube meets the lips / nostrils by using the numbers listed on the side of the ET tube				
12.	Secured the ET tube by adhesive tape and cleaned the area above the cuff of secretions by gently suctioning deep in to the oropharynx				
13.	Repeated pharyngeal suctioning				
	Evaluation				
1.	Alarm kept on				
2.	Emergency equipment such as a hand held resuscitation bag kept ready				
	Recording and reporting				
1.	Recorded in the nurses notes and on the respiratory flow sheet the point where the tube is placed and procedure done by whom date and time mode of ventilator setting				
2.	Reported to physician about significant readings				

Signature of Student --

Signature of Clinical Instructor --------------------------------

Performance Evaluation: Monitoring Client with Temporary Cardiac Pacemaker Support

Cardiac pacemaker, an electric apparatus used for maintaining a normal sinus rhythm of myocardial apparatus, used for maintaining a normal sinus rhythm of myocardial contraction by electrically stimulating the heart muscle. When the heart does not spontaneously contract at a minimum rate.

Sl. No.	Performance Criteria	S	U	NP	Comments
	Assessment				
1.	Identified the client who is receiving temporary cardiac pacemaker support				
2.	Discussed the terms pertinent to pacemaker therapy				
3.	Identified the routes used for temporary internal pacemakers				
4.	Differentiates between unipolar and bipolar electrodes				
	Implementation				
1.	Identified and intervenes appropriately when the following complications occurs, failure to pace, failure to capture and failure to sense				
2.	Changes the dressing over the insertion site				
3.	Initiates appropriate electrical safety precautions				
4.	Changes the pacemaker battery routinely				
5.	Perform an atrial electrocardiogram (AEG) with the atrial epicardial wires as directed				
	Recording and reporting				
1.	Documents all pertinent information				
2.	Report to the physician any significant changes				

Signature of Student -------------------------------------

Signature of Clinical Instructor ------------------------------

Performance Evaluation: Client with Cardiac Monitoring

Sl. No.	Performance Criteria	S	U	NP	Comments
	Assessment				
1.	Identified client requiring cardiac monitoring				
2.	Obtains a baseline heart rate and blood pressure				
	Implementation				
1.	Obtains and interprets a baseline rhythm strip every 4 hourly				
2.	Auscultate the heart sounds				
3.	Assessed the skin for color, temperature, turgor, edema and diaphoresis				
4.	Inspected nail bed for capillary refilling				
5.	Palpated the peripheral arterial pulses				
6.	Inspects the internal jugular veins for distension				
7.	Assess the hemodynamic wave form				
8.	Set alarm limits according to hospital policy				
9.	Institutes advanced cardiac life support as ordered				
10.	Obtains 12 leads ECG				
11.	Distinguish artifact an electrical (60 cycle) interference from the client				
	Evaluation				
1.	Observed for • Disturbance in impulse formation • Cardiac arrhythmias • Disturbance in impulse conduction				
2.	Prepared the client for the transfer from the monitor to the unmonitored state				
	Recording and reporting				
1.	Recorded pertinent information in nurses notes				
2.	Informed physician significant changes				

Signature of Student ---------------------------------------

Signature of Clinical Instructor --------------------------------

Performance Evaluation: Recording an Electrocardiogram (ECG)

Sl. No.	Performance Criteria	S	U	NP	Comments
	Assessment				
1.	Verified ECG requirement				
2.	Asked female patients to remove all tight fitting clothing around the chest				
3.	Checked ECG machine is in working condition				
4.	Ensured that the machine is properly earthed				
5.	Instructed the patient to lie relaxed in supine position				
	Nursing diagnosis				
1.	Health seeking behavior				
	Planning				
1.	Identified expected outcomes				
2.	Explained reasons for ECG recording				
3.	Provided privacy				
	Implementation				
1.	Explained procedure to the client				
2.	Prepared the chest, (shaving may be required in case of male patient) applied electro conductive gel on lead placement sites and placed all electrodes appropriately				
3.	Placed electrodes appropriately • V 1- 4th intercostals space right to sternum • V 2- 4th intercostals on the left side to sternum • V 3 –between V2 and V4 • V 4- 5th intercostals in midclavicular line • V 5- 5th intercostals space in the anterior auxillary line • V 6- 5th intercostals space in the mid auxillary line				
4.	Positioned the client as required by ensuring proper contact between the lead and skin				
5.	Recorded the ECG				
6.	Checked the ECG record for appropriateness and presence of artifacts				
7.	Removed electrodes, wiped the gel using tissue paper				
8.	Assisted patient in dressing				
9.	Replaced ECG machine				

Contd...

Contd...

Sl. No.	Performance Criteria	S	U	NP	Comments
10.	Labeled in ECG and pasted on ECG card				
11.	Sent ECG to physician for interpretation				
	Evaluation				
1.	Observed for significant changes in ECG, informed client to report to physician and follow up				
	Documentation				
1.	Recorded in ECG register. Informed sister incharge about procedure and report				

Signature of Student ---------------------------------------

Signature of Clinical Instructor -------------------------------

Performance Evaluation: Assisting with Lumbar Puncture

Sl. No.	Performance Criteria	S	U	NP	Comments
	Assessment				
1.	Determined purpose of the L.P.				
2.	Observed client alertness and awareness of surroundings				
3.	Observe for contraindication				
4.	Checked client history for allergies to local anesthetics, antiseptic solutions and iodine				
	Nursing diagnosis				
1.	• Anxiety related to lumber puncture procedure • Pain actual or potential related to lumber puncture				
	Planning				
1.	• The client cooperates and follow instructions during the procedure • The client receives no injury or untoward responses during procedure				
	Implementation				
1.	Explained the purpose and process of the procedure				
2.	Instructed the client to void before the procedure				
3.	Provided privacy where the procedure is done				

Contd...

Contd...

Sl. No.	Performance Criteria	S	U	NP	Comments
4.	Washed hands				
5.	Assessed the client vital signs				
6.	Assisted and instructed the client to remove clothing and lie on the examination table or bed. Covered with a drape				
7.	Positioned the client laterally with back at the edge of the table or bed				
8.	Drawn the client knees up to abdomen and flex chin toward chest				
9.	Placed all equipment on a table within the physician reach				
10.	Asked the patient to take deep breath				
11.	Asked the supporting staff to hold the client arms and legs in position				
12.	Handled supplies and equipment to the physician as required				
13.	Collected specimen container and labeled as indicated				
14.	Covered the client and assisted to a flat supine position for 12 hours or as required				
	Evaluation				
1.	Assessed needle insertion site for drainage				
2.	Assessed level of consciousness, vital signs, pupils, respiratory status, numbness or tingling in legs				
3.	Recorded and reported data in nurses notes				
4.	Reported pertinent findings to nurse incharge and clinical teacher				

Signature of Student ---------------------------------------

Signature of Clinical Instructor ------------------------------

CHAPTER

12

Nursing Assessment of Cardiovascular System

Name of the nursing institute --

Student name --

Specialty posting ---------------------Period from---------------to--------------

Nursing History

Demographic Data

Name of the patient	IP No.
Age	Gender
Marital status	Nationality
Language spoken	Religion
Occupation	Home town/city
Education	Income
Date of admission	Treatment received on arrival to hospital
Provisional diagnosis	Name of the doctor who is treating the patient ---------- -------------------- And unit ----------------------------

Date of Admission ------------------------------

Reason for visit --

When did the symptoms started---

General state of health ---

Was the onset sudden or gradual ---

How often the problem occurs --

Has the problem occur before --

Document the progression of the first manifestation--------------------------------

Chief Complaint

History of Present Illness

Ask any or all of the following as appropriate and write a summary.

Chief Complaint

Rely on objective testing (laboratory values).
Chest pain is one of the most common manifestations of cardiac disease.

Expanded Cardiac Assessment

Onset of chest pain	
Location	
Duration	
Characteristics	
Associated manifestation	Gastrointestinal disorders, like,burning/colic, aching, tightness Musculoskeletal disorders Aching Neurological disorders Aching/constant, burning, needle sharp Psychogenic states Vague burning/diffuse
Chest pain, typical pressure burning/heaviness/gradual onset • Worsened by • Exertion • Eating • Emotion • Cold • Deep breathing • Position changes • Relieved by • Rest • Nitroglycerin • Pain pills • Spontaneously	

Palpitation
- Specific review of systems
- Past medical history---
- Thyroid disease---
- Valvular heart disease---
- Heart murmur---
- Rheumatic heart disease--
- Medication prescription/ cold medications/nasal spray/ habits illicit drug use/caffeine intake.

Cyanosis
- Central /peripheral/unilateral/bilateral
- Congenital heart disease
- Pulmonary disease
- Tobacco use

Past medical history
- Childhood infectious disease
- Immunizations
- Hospitalizations
- Major illness/infectious disease
- Prior history of rheumatic fever
- Streptococcal infection
- Congenital abnormalities
- Previous hospitalization
- Outcome treatment

Allergies
- Environmental
- Food
- Medication
- Iodine/or contrast dye

Medication History
- Prescription
- Over the counter medication
- Vitamins-------------------------------
- Herbal--------------------------------
- Aspirin---------------------------
- Nitroglycerin-------------------------
- Laxatives-----------------------
- Nasal spray -----------------------

Dietary Habits
- Restriction advised yes/no
- Cholesterol/salt/fluid/sugar/caffeine intake

Family History

- Cardiovascular disease
- Hypertension
- Diabetes mellitus
- Stroke
- Renal disease
- Liver disease
- Relationship to member affected and treatment provided --

Physical Examination

Assessment Proceed from Head to Toe

General Appearance

General appearance

- Does the client lie, quietly/restless
- Position, lie flat/upright/erect position
- Respiratory distress/cyanosis/pallor/dyspnea

Patient general level of consciousness

- Client behavior appropriate for surroundings
- Fear/depression/anger
- Identify significant others
- Identify time

Vital signs

Temperature ---------------------

Respiration ---------- breath easily /does the client have to sit up to breath easily yes/no

Weight -------------------

Blood pressure, while client, lying-------------------sitting-------------standing----------

Pulse. Apical --------------radial ---------------tachycardia >100 beats/min/ Bradycardia <60 beats/min/iiregular pulse/bounding pulse/ absent pulse/tachypnea

Head and neck

- Eyes: A light gray ring around the iris (possibly caused by cholesterol deposits)
- Examine ear lobes normal. yes/no
- Lips and buccal mucosa normal. yes/no

Neck vein assessment

- Jugular vein. Engorges/slight provocation/distention absent with client at 45 degree angle

Abdomen

- Ascites /hyperactive bowel sounds/hypoactive bowel sounds

Skin • Central cyanosis/peripheral cyanosis/decreased turgor/warm to touch/cool to touch/edema
Nail • Clubbing/splinter hemorrhage

Diagnostic Testing

Diagnostic procedures are both noninvasive and invasive

Nursing responsibilities for these various tests include:

1. Scheduling the procedures
2. Explaining the purpose and the procedure and answering the any question
3. Procure consent
4. Providing prescribed medication for preprocedure
5. Providing physical and psychological support
6. Providing post procedure care

Noninvasive Tests

Name of the test	Test result
Electrocardiography tests	
Holter monitoring	
Exercise testing (tread meal test)	
Echocardiography	
Up right tilt table tests	
Radiographic cardiac tests	
Chest X-ray	
CT angiography	
CT scan pulmonary embolus protocol	
Magnetic resonance imaging	
Magnetic resonance angiography	
Visibility scan (positron emission tomography	

Invasive Cardiac Test

Transesophageal echocardiography	
Cardiac catheterization	
Left heart catheterization	
Right heart catheterization	

Contd...

Contd...

Electrophysiological studies	
Coronary angiography	
Hemodynamic monitoring	Arterial blood pressure --------------------------- --- Pulmonary artery pressure------------------- Pulmonary artery wedge pressure -----------

Clinical Performance Evaluation: Cardiovascular System

Perform a cardiovascular assessment

Sl. No.	Competency statement/criteria	Satisfactory = 1	Not satisfactory = 0	Not done
1.	Obtains a baseline heart rate (HR) and blood pressure (BP)			
2.	Obtains and interprets a baseline cardiac rhythm strip			
3.	Auscultates the heart sounds			
4.	Assesses the skin for color, temperature, turgor, edema, and diaphoresis			
5.	Inspect the nail bed for capillary refill			
6.	Palpates the peripheral arterial pulses			
7.	Inspects the internal jugular veins for distension			
8.	Assesses for the presence of central lines			
9.	Assesses the hemodynamic waveforms			
10.	Identifies the presence of a permanent or temporary pacemaker			

Signature of Student-----------------------------

Signature of Clinical Instructor-------------------

CHAPTER

13

Nursing Assessment of Respiratory System

Name of the nursing institute --

Student name --

Specialty posting ---------------------------Period from----------------to---------------

Nursing History

Demographic Data

Name of the Patient	IP No.
Age	Gender
Marital status	Nationality
Language spoken	Religion
Occupation	Home town/city
Education	Income
Date of admission	Treatment received on arrival to hospital
Provisional diagnosis	Name of the Doctor who is treating the patient -------- ---------------------- And unit ----------------------------

Date of admission ------------------------------

Reason for visit ---

When did the symptoms started--

General state of health ---

Was the onset sudden or gradual --

How often the problem occurs --

Has the problem occur before --

Document the progression of the first manifestation-----------------------------------

Chief Complaint

History of Present Illness

Ask any or all of the following as appropriate and write a summary

---

Chief Complaint

Rely on objective testing (laboratory values) Breathing pattern changed	
Unexplained restlessness or irritability	
Dyspnea (shortness of breath)	
Wheezing	
Pleuritic chest pain	
Tachycardia	
Cough	
Sputum production	
Hemoptysis	
Voice change	
Cyanosis	
Diaphoresis	
Decreased urinary output	

Respiratory History

Assessment	What type of breathing problems are you having--------------------------------------- Describe the problem you are having with your heart -------------------------------------- Does it occur a specific time of the day, during or after exercise, or all the time--- How has your breathing pattern changed --- Are you having sputum with coughing? Is the different------------------------------------- Are you having any chest pain? Does the pain occur with breathing---------------------- When did you notice your sputum change in color and amount Have you been exposed to cold or flu-------

Contd...

Contd...

Breathing pattern changed related to activities	
Cigarette smoking history	Are you smoking—yes/no If yes. how many cigarette each day -------- Since how long ------------------------- Are you interested in stopping—yes/no Have you ever smoked any drugs—yes/no Breathlessness—nothing at all /very slight/moderate/severe/ very severe Are you ever short of breath during exercise/at rest—yes/no

Past medical history

- Childhood infectious disease-------------------------------
- Immunizations-----------------------------
- Hospitalizations------------------
- Major illness/infectious disease-----------------
- Prior history of rheumatic fever------------------
- Streptococcal infection-----------------------
- Congenital abnormalities---------------------
- Previous hospitalization--------------------
- Outcome treatment-------------------------

Allergies

- Environmental
- Food
- Medication
- Iodine/or contrast dye

Medication history

- Prescription------------------------
- Over the counter-------------------
- Vitamins----------------------------
- Herbal------------------------------
- Bronchodilators -------------------
- Nasal spray -------------------------

Dietary habits

- Restriction advised—yes/no
- Have you recently lost weight—yes/no
- Do any particular foods affect your sputum production or breathing----
----

Family history

- Patient received immunization for influenza
- Any of the family member suffered with—wheeze/strider/(continuous musical sound constant pitch) absent breath sounds/ COPD/ TB/ Lung cancer

Physical Examination

Assessment proceed from head to toe

General appearance

General appearance
- Does the client lie, quietly/restless
- Position, lie flat/upright/erect position
- Respiratory distress/cyanosis/pallor/dyspnea

Patient general level of consciousness
- Client behavior appropriate for surroundings
- Fear/depression/anger
- Identify significant others
- Identify time

Vital signs
Temperature ---------------------
Respiration ---------- breath easily/does the client have to sit up to breath easily yes/no
Weight -------------------
Blood pressure. while client, lying--------------------sitting--------------standing-----------
Pulse. Apical --------------radial ---------------tachycardia >100 beats/min/Bradycardia < 60 beats/min/irregular pulse/bounding pulse/ absent pulse/tachyapnea

CHAPTER

14

Assessment of Community Health Nursing

Evaluation Tool for Community Health Nursing Experience

Name of the student: --------------------------- Year of study ---------------------------

Batch: --------------------Name of community area: --------------------------

Sl. No.	Criteria	Excellent	Very good	Good	Satisfactory	Poor
	Cognitive skills	4	3	2	1	0
1.	Follows principles of community health nursing					
2.	Understands the individuals, families, and significant others					
3.	Identifies the demographic characteristics					
4.	Exhibits skills in history taking and physical examination of individuals and families					
5.	Diagnosis the community health needs of the individuals					
	Technical skills					
6.	Demonstrate home visit technique during home visit					
7.	Identifies the demographic characteristics and collect data					
8.	Collect vital statistics					

Contd...

Contd...

Sl. No.	Criteria	Excellent	Very good	Good	Satisfactory	Poor
9.	Collect history and exhibits skills in physical examination if needed					
10.	Provides family welfare services					
11.	Refer the individuals or family to appropriate referral center if needed					
	Professional conduct					
12.	Always well groomed and neat, conscious, about professional appearance					
13.	Punctual, never been late					
14.	Courteous and considerate towards others					
15.	Identifies and accepts the beliefs and practices of others including patient's family and community					
16.	Listens to individuals, family, community, coworker and seniors					
17.	Communicate with various national and international agencies					
18.	Encourage active participation of family and community in their own health activities					
19.	Participate in national health program					

Contd...

Contd...

Sl. No.	Criteria	Excellent	Very good	Good	Satisfactory	Poor
	Health education					
20.	Identifies needs for health education					
21.	Provides health education as per needs of individuals, family and community					
	Records and reports					
22.	Knows to who the information to be communicated					
23.	Records and reports patients information accurately					
24.	Use appropriate language					
25.	Decides on specific information to bc communicated					

Rating Scale

4 = Excellent, 3 = Very Good, 2 = Good, 1 = Average, 0 = Poor.

Grade

Above 110 = Excellent
91 – 100 = Very good
81 – 90 = Good
71 – 80 = Satisfactory
61 – 70 = Poor

Signature of the Student ----------

Signature of the Teacher in-charge ---------- **Signature of HOD ----------**

Family Profile/Family Folder and Health Record

Name of the community area: Rural/urban --

Student's name --Year of study ------------------

Date of commencement of study-----------------Date of completion-----------------

Name of the health center--

Family identification

- Name of the head of the family--
- Address --
- Occupation ----------------------------Contact number ---------------------------------
- Religion -----------------Type of family, nuclear/joint/extended
- Education ------------------------Total income of the family ----------------------------

Family Composition

Sl. No.	Name of the members	Relationship with head of the family	Age	Sex	Education occupation	Income	Health status

Housing and sanitary condition

Type of house—Kutcha/Pucca/ Semipucca /tiles . Own/ Rented
Numbers of rooms-------------------------- No. of inhabitants --------------------------
Sleeping arrangements--------------------Provision of privacy: Yes/no
Ventilation: Adequate/inadequate/no ventilation
When was the house sprayed last –date-------------- If no state reason--------------------
Facilities for personal cleanliness/bathing: Adequate/inadequate
Living space: Adequate/inadequate
Lighting: Electricity/gas lamp/oil lamp
Drinking water supply: Public supply/bore well/open well/open tank
Kitchen ventilation and light: Adequate/inadequate.
For cooking use fire wood/gas/kerosene/cow dung
Toilets type: Sanitary/use public lavatory/open air defecation
Cloth washing facilities: Adequate/use tank water/open well
Drainage system: Open/closed/ soakage/drain/kitchen garden/pit.
Is the sullage water being disposed hygienically: Yes/ no.
Measure to control insects, flies, and rodents. present/ no measures
System of waste disposal (disposed hygienically if yes say, close to the house /separate from the house/separate from residence area (burning/ burying/composing)

Contd...

Contd...

Housing and sanitary condition
Open space around the house: Yes/no. Water stagnation: Yes/no Are the cattle and poultry housed hygienically: Seperate/within house Is there a well or hand pump Is it maintained in good order? Yes/no. When was the well chlorinated (date) – state reasons for not chlorinated Are there any stray dogs in the vicinity: Yes/no. If yes, write approximate number of dogs--- Cultural background. Belief about health practices-- Summary (any relevant information)---

Family health status
Regular screening for health practice. Followed/not followed Dental check up practiced/not practiced Any members of the family suffering from chronic fever. if yes write name, age, diagnosis (if known) treatment receiving--- Does any member have a cough for more than two weeks -- Does any one have skin disease (e.g. itching, patch, rash) if yes write name, age, diagnosis and treatment --- Does any one have any other illness (Dengu,STD, HIV). If yes write detail--- Is there any family history of asthma/cancer/diabetes/epilepsy/hypertension/heart disease/ hepatitis/hemophilia/stroke/tuberculosis/mental disorders/Thyroid or autoimmune disorders aged grand parent and siblings alive? If so what is there current state of health if not state the cause of death and age of death

Food consumption by the family members (calculate for one day or one week). Note based on the total family income able to meet caloric requirements

Sl. No.	Breakfast	Midmorning	Lunch	Evening snacks	Dinner	Total intake of Carbohydrates-------- Protein--------- Fat-------------

Note selection and preparation of food---

Any family members suffering from malnutrition. If yes take complete nutrition assessment ---

Assessment---

Is there any child under five in family who shows signs of malnutrition?

Sl. No.	Name	Age	Kwashiorkor	Marasmus	Vitamin A deficiency	Anemia	Rickets

Summary ---

Sleep and Rest
Sleep disturbance in any members in the family-- Sleep pattern of family members--

Vital Statistics

Birth Details

Sl. No.	Date of birth	Sex	Parent's name	Remarks

Death Details

Sl. No.	Date of death	Sex	Parent's name	Remarks

Marriages Details

Sl. No.	Names	Age	Date of marriage	Remarks
Bride				
Bridegroom				

Under Five Children
Immunization status of under five children -- Specify name, age, and reason for not being immunized--------------------------------------- --- • BCG vaccination • DPT vaccination • Poliomyelitis vaccination • Measles vaccination • Vit A solution

Eligible couple
Is there any eligible couple. If yes, list their name --

Sl. No.	Name of the couple	Age	Using a contraceptive method	Vasectomy	Tubal legation	Oral contraceptive

Specify if any couple not interested to adopt FP method (state the reason)

Using contraceptive method. If yes specify: Vasectomy/tubal ligation ----------
----

Is any woman pregnant if yes, write the following remarks

1. Gravida ---------------------------
2. Registered in the hospital: Yes/no
3. Pregnant women receiving iron and folic acid: Yes/no
4. Women receiving tetanus toxid----------------------

Vulnerable family members--

Sl. No.	Vulnerable family members	Name of the family members	Number	Health assessment	Problem identified
1.	Under 5 children				
2.	Antenatal mothers				
3.	Lactating mothers				
4.	School children				
5.	Adolescent				
6.	Elderly				
7.	Challenged physically and mentally				
8.	Others				

Transport and communication media
Transport: Owns/tempo/tractor/uses private transport
Telephone facilities: Yes/no.
Radio: Yes/no.
Newspaper/magazine: Yes/no
Postal service/telegraph facilities. Yes/no
Language known----------------------------------

Dietary Pattern

Basic food practice in the family	Food used	Traditional	Ideal	Unhygienic
Rice				
Jawar				
Wheat				
Vegetable				
Fish				
Meat				
Egg				
Milk and milk product				
Pulses				
Tubers				

Statement of the Expenditure of the Family

Sl. No.	Items	Amount spent on each item	Percentage of amount spent on each item
1.	Food		
2.	Clothing		
3.	Housing: Rent, if own house, other utility expenditure		
4.	Medicine regular or any systemic disease in the members (like diabetes, hypertension, etc.)		
5.	Children education		
6.	Recreation		
7.	Smoking or liquor		
8.	Debt		
9.	Savings		
10.	Others (specify)		

In addition, students are expected to obtain following information by observation and other methods

1. Description of the community location
2. Topography
3. Climate

4. History
5. No. of school
6. No. of healthcare agencies
7. Balwadi or ICDS Centers
8. Places of worship
9. Maintain record of road to health card for knowing degree of malnutrition for under 5 (use nutritional assessment).

Date of survey | Name and signature of the student

Signature of HOD | Signature of Principal

Home Visit Responsibility

Sl. No.	Responsibility	Task
1.	Pre-visit preparation	• Identify exact location of home • Prepare for safe visit
2.	Orientation period	• Introduce yourself • Review available family data • Identify family problems
3.	Intervention period	• Assess family needs/problem assessment • Suggest what need to be done as per health need so the family refer appropriately if needed • Give health teaching/counseling as needed • Assess need for other services • Any illness in the family/treatment receiving /advise as required
4.	Termination period	• Summarize visit activities with family member/ individual • Explain next visit

CHAPTER

15

Medical Surgical Nursing: Clinical Assessment Format

Teacher Instructions for Use of Clinical Assessment Form

Description of the Form

There are four major areas of student performance being measured with this form, nursing knowledge, medical knowledge, case studies, and professional conduct. Each area identifies certain standards which must be met in order for the student to achieve the highest marks for that standard, is the optimum behavior expected of the student.

Administration of the Form

1. This clinical assessment form is to be explained to the student at the beginning of the clinical experience in which it will be used.
2. The clinical assessment forms is to be completed by the clinical teacher at the end of clinical posting.
3. At the end of clinical experience, the completed form is to be discussed with the student and an explanation provided for any marks that are not understood by the student.
4. The student's signature on the form only indicate that the she/he has been presented with the form. If the student disagrees with the marking, the student should write a comment on the form to that effect and may persue the matter with the coordinator, or with the principal.

Use of the Form

1. Each standard has a four point rating scale with the following definitions
   Standard met: The student achieved all of the items identified in the standard.
   Standard almost met: The student achieved more than half of the items identified in the standard.
   Standard far from met: The student achieved less than half of the items identified in the standard.
   Standard not met: The student did not achieve the items identified in the standard.
2. Each standard has different marks depending on the importance of that standard to the overall assessment. The number of marks to be awarded for each point of the rating scale is listed in under that point.

Medical Surgical Nursing: Clinical Assessment Criteria

Students name---

Medical surgical unit --

Student's number--Ward--------------------- -------------------------From-------------------------------------to------------------------

Performance Level

Sl. No.	Standard	SM (3 M)	SAM (2 M)	SFFM (1 M)	SNM (0 M)	SNM
1.	**Nursing knowledge assessment and nursing diagnosis**					
A.	Collect thorough knowledge about patient illness					Unable to collect data about patient or has no knowledge about patient
B.	Recognizes the physical needs of the patient					Unable to assess patient physically. Needs constant guidance
C.	Identifies psychological needs of the patient and family					Unable to Identifies psychological needs of the patient and family
D.	Categorizes the patient problems					Unable to formulate complete nursing diagnosis
E.	Formulates complete nursing diagnosis					Unable to formulate complete diagnosis
2.	**Planning**					
A.	Prioritizes the patient needs					Unable to identify the prioritize needs

Contd...

Contd...

Sl. No.	Standard	SM (3 M)	SAM (2 M)	SFFM (1 M)	SNM (0 M)	SNM
B.	Establishes suitable nursing actions for each patient's needs					Unable to plan nursing actions for patient or unable to cope with routine work
C.	Able to organize nursing actions within the given time					Need more guidance and time to plan the nursing care
D.	Formulates the needed patient health instructions					Makes no attempt to find out the health learning needs of the patient and family
3.	**Implementation**					
A.	Competent in implementing nursing care thorough, safe and accurate, collects and replaces equipment, organizes activities within time					Demonstrate minimal competence in implementing nursing care. Disorganized, wastes time and energy. Rarely completes work within time
B.	Maintains comfortable environment for patient					Ignores body alignment. Doesn't pay attention to patient discomfort
C.	Applies scientific principles					Ignores scientific principles when carrying out care
D.	Maintains safe therapeutic environment					Unable to maintain healthy, safe and clean environment
E.	Accurately records and reports patient information					Fails to report or record accurate information

Contd...

Contd...

Sl. No.	Standard	SM (3 M)	SAM (2 M)	SFFM (1 M)	SNM (0M)	SNM
F.	Able to give planned health instructions to patient and family					Unable to give even incidental teaching to patient and family
4.	**Evaluation**					
A.	Establishes outcome criteria for the patient including physical state and behavior					Unable to set the outcome criteria or unable to monitor patient's progress
B.	Rationale: Able to state rationale for nursing actions					Unable to state rationale for nursing action
5.	**Medical knowledge**					
A.	Drug file presents written document as follows: Name of the drug, action, indications, dosage, ranges, contraindications, side effects, precautions					No written documentation of drugs administered
B.	Medical diagnosis: States accurate medical diagnosis of each patient cared for and describes etiology, signs and symptoms, medical therapy and results of medical therapy					Unable to state medical diagnosis(es) of each patient cared for nor describe etiology, signs and symptoms, medical therapy and results of therapy
C.	Laboratory investigation: States proper names of laboratory investigations of each patient cared for and describe reasons for tests, patient preparation for tests, test procedure					Unable to state name of laboratory investigations of each patient cared for nor describe reasons for tests, patient preparation or test procedure
D.	Case study: Accurately completes all sections of written case study format and submits on time					Does not present accurate written case study on time

Contd...

Contd...

Sl. No.	Standard	SM (3 M)	SAM (2 M)	SFFM (1 M)	SNM (0 M)	SNM
6.	**Professional conduct**					
A.	Uniform: Always well groomed and neat, conscious about professional appearance					Pays no attention to grooming and is untidy
B.	Punctuality: Exceptionally punctual for clinical and has never been late, completes all learning assignments on time					Consistently late for clinical, makes no attempt to complete the given learning assignments on time, stops in mid task when clinical hours are over
C.	Sense of responsibility: Readily accpects responsibility, reliable, adaptable and displays consistency in work, judgement is consistently sound and logical, works effectively under pressure					Reluctant to take responsibility and avoids it. Likely to make illogical hasty decisions and tends to lose control under excessive pressure
D.	Initiative for self learning : Eager to learn and seek new learning experiences self directives in expanding knowledge and utilizing available resources and has original ideas					Fails to participate in new learning experiences or utilizing available resources to expand knowledge even when directed to do so. Lacks capacity for independent actions and always needs specific directions
7.	**Communication skill**					
A.	Patient and family: Establishes and maintains outstanding working relationships with patients and families					Fails to establishes effective working relationship with patients and families

Contd...

Contd...

Sl. No.	Standard	SM (3 M)	SAM (2 M)	SFFM (1 M)	SNM (0M)	SNM
B.	Hospital staff/health team: Establishes harmonious relationship with the members of the health team, deals with them skillfully, smoothly and with insight, polite and helpful					Has difficulty in getting along with other members of the health team and is argumentative
C.	Colleagues: Very well accepected by colleagues. Always concerned about them and works well with them					Not accepted by the colleagues, tends to remain alone. Demonstrate little interest in others
D.	Teachers: Always respects rules and regulations, accepts constructive criticism					Shows no respect for teachers. Breaks rules and regulations and resents constructive criticisms

Sub total of marks---------------------------------------

Total possible marks -----------------------Total marks obtained--------------------------

Signature of student---

Signature of teacher ---

Date signed --

Key

SM = standard met
SAM = standard almost met
SFFM = standard for from met
SNM = standard not met

Medical Surgical Nursing Case Study Assessment Criteria

Name of the student -----------------------------Medical surgical unit------------

Name of the hospital-----------------Area-----------Date of case study started-----

Date ended -----------------Name of the patient-----------Diagnosis----------------

Name of the clinical teacher in-charge---

Sl. No.	Criteria	Excellent	Good	Average	Satisfactory	Poor
1.	Assessment Obtain a baseline data and collect history					
2.	Perform a physical examination					
3.	Identifies basic needs of patients based on assessment and history					
4.	Understanding patient disease condition					
5.	Diagnosis Categorizes the patients needs/problems					
6.	Formulates nursing diagnosis as per priority					
7.	Planning Plans nursing actions for each needs of the patient					
8.	State the outcome criteria/ objectives					
9.	Involve patient and family members while planning					
10.	Prioritizes the patient needs					
11.	Implementation: Implements nursing care competently, safely, and accurately within a given time					
12.	Compare laboratory investigation and clinical findings with patients data					
13.	Follows nutritional requirements for patients , and compare the standard nutritional requirements					

Contd...

Contd...

Sl. No.	Criteria	Excellent	Good	Average	Satisfactory	Poor
14.	Maintains safe environment for patient and apply scientific principles					
15.	Records and reports patients information accurately					
16.	Follow the principles of drug administration					
17.	Compares, definition, etiology, signs and symptoms, pathophysiology, medical management, nursing management of disease condition with the text books (theoretical knowledge)					
18.	Gives health instructions to patient and family					
19.	Evaluation: Identifies outcome criteria used to evaluate the patients response to nursing care					
20.	Collects data related to identified criteria					
21.	Re-examine the patient's care plan					
22.	Modifies the care plan					
23.	Establishes and maintains outstanding working relationships					
24.	Include research study related to disease condition/ diagnosis of the patient					
	Bibliography					

Signature of Student

Signature of Clinical Supervisor
Signature of Principal

Score

Excellent = 5
Good = 4
Average = 3
Satisfactory = 2
Poor = 1

Medical Surgical Nursing Care Plan Evaluation

Name of the student --------------------------------Level of student----------------------

Name of the hospital------------Area-----------Date of case study started ----------

Date ended -------------Name of the patient-----------Diagnosis----------------------

Name of the clinical teacher incharge--

Sl. No.	Criteria	Excellent	Good	Average	Satisfactory	Poor
1.	**Assessment** Obtain a baseline data and collect history					
2.	Perform a physical examination					
3.	Identifies basic needs of patients based on assessment and history					
4.	Understanding patient disease condition					
5.	Diagnosis Categorizes the patients needs/problems					
6.	Formulates nursing diagnosis as per priority					
7.	**Planning** Plans nursing actions for each needs of the patient					
8.	State the outcome criteria/ objectives					
9.	Involve patient and family members while planning					
10.	Prioritizes the patient needs					
11.	**Implementation** Implements nursing care competently, safely, and accurately within a given time					
12.	Compare laboratory investigation and clinical findings with patients data					
13.	Maintains safe environment for patient and apply scientific principles					

Contd...

Contd...

Sl. No.	Criteria	Excellent	Good	Average	Satisfactory	Poor
14.	Records and reports patients information accurately					
15.	Follow the principles of drug administration					
16.	Gives health instructions to patient and family					
17.	**Evaluation** Identifies outcome criteria used to evaluate the patients response to nursing care					
18.	Collects data related to identified criteria					
19.	Re-examine the patient's care plan					
20.	Modifies the care plan					
21.	Establishes and maintains outstanding working relationships					
	Bibliography					

Signature of Student

Signature of Clinical Supervisor

Signature of Principal

Score

Excellent = 5
Good = 4
Average = 3
Satisfactory = 2
Poor = 1

CHAPTER

16

Nursing Assessment of Child Health

Guidelines for Developmental Screening

Why screen for disability?

It is important to detect disability early so that remedial measures can be undertaken to minimize their adverse effects on the child health. The disability can be detected by the routine screening of all children as part of the primary child care. It is generally agreed that early detection of disabilities leads to better prognosis.

Who should do the screening?

It is important to detect disabilities early so that remedial measures can be undertaken to minimize their adverse effects on the child's health. The disabilities can be detected by routine screening of all children as part of the primary child care.

Who should do the screening?

Developmental screening is the responsibility of all health care providers who see children. All concerned staff will be trained.

What is developmental screening?

This is a comparison of a child's responses and behaviors to what is normally expected of a child of that age. The following four biological characteristics are used as parameters for screening.

1. **Motor development:** Involving body posture and physical competence.
2. **Language development:** Involving ability to hear, listen, and to use speech.
3. **Cognitive development:** Involving processing and understanding of ideas and concepts.
4. **Social adaptive development:** Involving self identity, self help and acceptance of social behavior with regard to personal relationships.

Newborn Reflexes

1. Rooting reflex
2. Sucking reflex
3. Swallowing

4. Gagging
5. Sneezing and coughing
6. Extrusion
7. Blinking
8. Doll's eye
9. Palmar grasp
10. Plantar grasp
11. Dancing (step in place)
12. Babinski reflex
13. Tonic neck
14. Moro reflex

Child Health Assessment

History Taking and General Physical Examination

Name of the student-------------------------------------Course -----------------------

Date ------------------------ Clinical posting (specialty) -------------------------------

Child Health History

Informant's relationship to child --

Name of the child	IP No.
Age in months if under 3 years	Gender Ordinal position of the child
Language spoken	Nationality
Income of the parent	Religion
Education status (if school age child)	Home town/city Address
Date of admission	Reason for admission
Provisional diagnosis	Treatment received on arrival to hospital

Nursing history

Family: Home environment

Name	Age	Health status	Education	Occupation
Family members in home (that is, parents siblings, grand parents, others)				

Hereditary illness ---

Child

If both parents are working who take the care of the child	
Any significant vital statistics in the family	

Eating Behavior

Bottle-feed	
Breastfeed	
Cup or spoon. If cup or spoon is being used how is this being done	
Age of weaning. Type of formula	
Amount of milk per day	
Amount of water per day	
Feeding or eating problems	

Elimination

Number of bowel movements daily	
Use training chair	
Time taken to bathroom	
If toilet training is being done. Method used	
Problem regarding elimination	Diarrhea/constipation, incontenent urine/faces
Urinary stream/frequency of voiding	

Sleeping

Sleep in crib/bed/alone	Special bed time rituals
Usual bed time	
Fears for dark	
Problem related to sleep	
Nightmares	
Sleep walking	
Bed wetting	If yes, how handled

Personal Hygiene

Care by another	Dressing/brushing teeth
Need assistance with personal hygiene	
Problem related to personal hygiene	
Dental hygiene and problem	

Behavior

How does child react to distress?	Crying, temper tantrum, withdraw, runaway.
Disciplinary measure	
Behavior problems	If yes, how handled
Plays	Usually alone/parallel play/play activity and toys enjoyed

Handicaps

Vision	
Hearing	
Speech	
Dental	
Gait	
Other handicaps	
Supportive devices	
Communication and socialization	Problem with communication. Explain

Health History

Ask Any or All of the Following as Appropriate and Write Summary Below

What problem made to bring to hospital?	
When this symptoms started?	
Any precipitating factors/aggravating (what were you doing at that time)	
Was the onset sudden or gradual?	
How often does the problem occur?	
Where is the exact location of the problem?	
Has the problem occurred before?	
Significant area affected	
Direct admission	
Referred by others	

Any relevant information ---

Natal history	Gestation normal /deviation from normal
Birth	Normal /deviation from normal
How soon bonding taken place?	

Clinical Assessment Tool for Pediatrics Nursing

Student's name -----------------------------------Hospital----------------------------

Student's roll number----------------------------Ward--------------------------------

Instructor's name --

Posting from----------------------------to ---

Required clinical behaviors	Performance level= comments

Sl. No.	Required clinical behaviors	SM 3	SAM 2	AFFM 1	SNM 0	SNM= Comments
1.	**Nursing knowledge** A. Nursing Process. **Assessment and nursing diagnosis**					
1.1.	Collects the data about the child's needs (physical and psychological) during illness					Unable to collect the data about the child's needs (physical and psychological) during illness
1.2.	Assesses the child's growth and developmental needs					Unable to assess the child's growth and developmental needs
1.3.	Recognizes the psychosocial development stages					Recognizes the psychosocial development stages
1.4.	Assesses the nutritional needs of the child					Unable to assess the nutritional needs of the child
1.5.	Recognizes play needs of the child					Unable to recognize play needs of the child
1.6.	Assesses the child's parents and family members knowledge about the child condition					Unable to assess the child's parents and family members knowledge about the child condition
1.7.	Categorizes the child needs					Unable to categorize the child's needs
1.8.	Formulates nursing diagnoses					Unable to formulate nursing diagnoses

Contd...

Contd...

Sl. No.	Required clinical behaviors	SM 3	SAM 2	AFFM 1	SNM 0	SNM= Comments
2.	**Planning**					
2.1.	Prioritizes the child's needs according to the developmental stages of the child					Unable to identify the priority the child's needs according to the developmental stages of the child
2.2.	Establishes and recognizes for suitable nursing actions each child needs					Unable to establish and recognizes for suitable nursing actions each child needs
2.3.	Considers psychosocial needs of the child when planning nursing care					Unable to consider psychosocial needs of the child when planning nursing care
2.4.	Develops nutritional plan for the child					Unable to develop nutritional plan for the child
2.5.	Plan play needs					Unable to plan play needs
2.6.	Involves child, parents and family members in planning for health teaching					Unable to Involve child, parents and family members in planning for health teaching
3.	**Implementation**					
3.1.	Maintains safe ,and therapeutic environment according to developmental stage					Unable to maintain safe, and therapeutic environment according to developmental stage
3.2.	Thorough safe and accurate in implementing planned nursing care according to the child's needs					Unable to implement thorough safe and accurate in implementing planned nursing care according to the child's needs
3.3.	Meets nutritional needs of the child's as planned					Meets nutritional needs of the child's as planned

Contd...

Contd...

Sl. No.	Required clinical behaviors	SM 3	SAM 2	AFFM 1	SNM 0	SNM= Comments
3.4.	Meets play needs of the child					Unable to meet play needs of the child
3.5.	Gives planned health education to the child's parents and family members					Unable to give planned health education to the child's parents and family members
3.6.	Maintains accuracy and economy while giving care					Unable to maintain accuracy and economy while giving care
3.7.	Accurate in recording and reporting child's significant information to the appropriate personnel					Fails to report accurate and significant information to the appropriate personnel
4.	**Evaluation**					
4.1.	Evaluates with guidance the care given					Unable to evaluate the care even with guidance
4.2.	Modifies the plan					Unable to modify the plan
5.	**Medical knowledge**					
5.1.	**Medical diagnosis:** Know medical diagnosis of each child cared for and able to describe pathophysiology, predisposing factors, etiology, signs and symptoms, therapeutic management and results					No knowledge about medical diagnosis of child cared for and unable to describe pathophysiology, predisposing factors, etiology, signs and symptoms, therapeutic management and results
5.2.	**Investigations:** Describe investigations done and knows the reasons, preparation and procedures and interprets the result of the specific tests done for the child cared					Unable to describe Investigations done and does not knows the reasons and interprets the result of the various tests done for the child cared

Contd...

Contd...

Sl. No.	Required clinical behaviors	SM 3	SAM 2	AFFM 1	SNM 0	SNM= Comments
5.3.	Medications: Able to describe and calculate the drugs administered, knows the name, action, indications, dosage, toxic effect, precautions and presents written document, for the drugs administration					Unable to calculate the drug dosage did not present written. The documentation of any drug administers to the child care
6.	**Professional conduct**					
6.1.	**Uniform** Always well groomed and neat, conscious about professional appearance					Pay no attention to grooming and is untidy
6.2.	**Punctuality** Exceptionally punctual for clinical and has never been late, completes all given learning assignments on time					Consistently late for clinical. Makes no attempt to complete the given learning assignments on time. Stops in mid task when clinical hours over
6.3.	**Sense of responsibility** Readily accpects responsibilities, reliable, adaptable, and displays consistently in work, judgments is consistently sound and logical works effectively under pressure					Reluctant to take responsibility and avoids it, make illogical and avoids it. Hasty decisions and lends to lose control under excessive pressure
6.4.	**Initiate for self learning** Eager to learn and seek new learning experiences, self directive in expands knowledge and utilizing available resources and has original ideas					Fails to participate in new learning experience or in utilizing available resources to expand knowledge. Even when directed to do so. Lacks capacity for independent action and always needs specific directions

Contd...

Contd...

Sl. No.	Required clinical behaviors	SM 3	SAM 2	AFFM 1	SNM 0	SNM= Comments
6.5.	**Communication skills:** a. **Child and parents and families:** Establish and maintains outstanding working relationships with children and family members					Fails to establish effective working relationship with children and family members
	b. **Hospital staff and health team:** Establishes a harmonious relationship with the members of health team, deals with them skillfully, and with insight, polite and helpful					Has difficulty in getting along with other members of the health team and argumentative
	c. **Colleagues:** Very well accepted by colleagues. Always concerned about them and works well with them. Teachers: always respects rules and regulations. Accepts constructive criticism	4	4	2		Not accepted by the colleagues, tends to remain alone. Demonstrate little interest in others. Shows no respect for teachers, breaks rules and regulations as result does not accepts constructive criticism

Total marks = 100	**Marks obtained =**
Comments: Student's signature: Instructors signature: Date signed:	

Growth and Development Infancy to Adolescence

Age	Weight	Height
Infancy: Birth to 6 months	• Weekly gain 140 g to 200 g • Birth weight doubles by age 6 months	Monthly gain: (1") 2.5 cms
6 to 12 months	Weight gain 85–140 g (3–5 oz) Birth weight triples by age 12 months	Monthly gain: (1/2") 1.25 cm 50% over birth length by age 12 months
Toddler: 1 to 3 years	Yearly gain: (4 ½ to 6 ½ lbs) 2 to 3 kg Birth weight quadruples by age 2 ½	Yearly gain: (3" to 4") 7.5 to 10 cms
Preschool age: 3 to 6	Yearly gain: (4 ½ to 6 ½ lb) 2 to 3 kg	Yearly gain (2"to 3") 5 to 7 cm Birth length doubles by age 4
School age 6 to 12	Yearly gain: (4 ½ to 6 ½ lbs) 2 to 3 kg	Yearly gain: (2") 5 cm
Adolescence: 13 to 21 years	Females: Highly variable; gain of (15 to 55 lbs). Over a period of 3b years b7 to 25 kg Growth spurt begins at average age of 11 Males: Highly variable; gain of (15 to 65 lbs) 7 to 30 kg Growth spurt begins at average age of 13	Females: Highly variable; gain of (2" to 10") 5 to 25 cm Males: Highly variable; gain of (4" to 12") 10 to 30 cms

Time of Eruption and Shedding of Primary Teeth

Name	Eruption of tooth age in months		Shedding of tooth age in year	
	Lower	Upper	Lower	Upper
Central incisor	6	7-1/2	6	7-1/2
Lateral incisor	7	9	7	8
Cuspid	16	18	9-1/2	11-1/2
First molar	12	14	10	10-1/2
Second molar	20	24	11	10-1/2

Incisors range ± 2 months
Molars range ± 4 months

Time of Eruption of Permanent Teeth

Name	Lower age in years	Upper age in years
Central incisors	6–7	7–8
Lateral incisors	7–8	8–9
Cuspid	9–10	11–12
First bicuspids	10–12	10–11
Second bicuspids	11–12	10–12
First molars	6–7	6–7
Second molars	11–13	12–13
Third molars	17–21	17–21

National Immunization Schedule

Age	Vaccine	Dosage	Route of administration
At birth	BCG for institutional deliveries OPU zero dose (for institutional deliveries)	0.05 mL 2 drops	Intradermal Oral
6 weeks	BCG if not given at birth	0.05 mL	Intradermal
	DPT 1	0.5 mL	Deep intramuscular
	OPV 1	2 drops /0.5 mL	Oral
10 weeks	DPT 2	0.5 mL	Deep intramuscular
	OPV 2	2 drops	Oral
14 weeks	DPT 3	0.5 mL	Deep IM
	OPV 3	2 drops	2 drops
9 months	MMR	0.5 mL	Subcutaneous
16–24 months	DPT (booster dose)	0.5 mL	Subcutaneous
	OPV (booster dose)	2 drops	Oral
5 to 6 years	DT (A second dose of DT after 4 weeks if no evidence of previous immunization with DPT)	0.5 mL	Deep IM

Contd...

Contd...

Age	Vaccine	Dosage	Route of administration
10 to 16 Years	Tetanus toxoid (A second dose of TT after 4 weeks if no evidence of previous immunization with DPT, DT, or TT)	0.5 mL	Deep IM
For pregnant women	TT 1 in early pregnancy TT 2 after 4 weeks	0.5 mL	Intramuscular

As per Extended Program of Immunization

Booster doses OPV		19 months	Oral	0.5 mL 5 drops
DPT + Oral polio		16–24 months		
DT		5 Years		
Tetanus toxid		At 10 years and again at 16 years		

Vitamin A. Supplementation has been integrated into extended program of immunization (EPI) 9,18, 24, 30 and 36 months.

Vitamin A 100,000 IU are given with measles dose at 9 months and Vitamin A 200,000 IU are given with MMR dose at 15 months.

Mothers given vitamin A 200,000 IU immediately after delivery or within 15 days after delivery. Mother is given one dose only of rubella.

(Vaccine storage requirement: Temperature range: + 20°C to + 80°C).

Abbreviations

BCG = Bacillus Calmittee Gurein
DPT = Diphtheria, Pertussia and Tetanus
OPV= Oral Polio Vaccine
DT = Diphtheria and Tetanus Vaccine.

Additional Vaccination

6 weeks	H.Influenza B
10 weeks	H.Influenza B
14 weeks	H.Influenza B
18 months	H.Influenza B
15–18 months	Mumps, measles, rubella (MMR)
24 months	Typhoid

Assessment of Infant

Sl. No.	Criteria/activities	As per text / theory	Infant picture	Remarks
1.	**Anthropometric measurements**			
	Height			
	Weight			
	Chest circumference			
	Head circumference			
2.	**Vital signs**			
	Respiration			
	Pulse			
	Temperature			
3.	**Gross motor development**			
	Head control			
	Roll over back	2 months		
	Sit with support	4 months		
	Sit without support	4 months		
	Pull to sit from supine position	6 months		
	Pull to stand	6 months		
	Creeps	10 months		
	Crawls on belly	9 months		
	Cruises (walks sideways by holding and supporting object)	10 months		
	Stepping movements	6 months		
	Stand without support	12 months		
	Walk a few steps	12 months		
	Walk	12 months		
4.	**Fine motor and adoptive development**			
	Eye coordination			
	Follows an object with an unsteady movements of the eye ball	2 months		

Contd...

Contd...

Sl. No.	Criteria/activities	As per text / theory	Infant picture	Remarks
	Follows on object with steady movements of the eye ball and able to focus	2 months		
	Hand eye coordination			
	Pincer finger thumb fine grasp to pick up a pellet	5 months		
	Able to grasp colored object	4 months		
	Able to hold some toys	4 months		
	Hand mouth coordination	4 months		
	Try to feed with spillage			
5.	**Emotional and social development**			
	Social smile	2 months		
	Enjoys in watching his image in a mirror	9 months		
	Shows some resistance while removing a toy from him	5 months		
	Put some effort to get a toy which is kept out of his reach	5 months		
	Stranger anxiety	7 months		
	Solitary play	12 months		
	Begins to play peek a boo`	10 months		
6.	**Language development**			
	Watches mother intently when she speaks to him	2 months		
	Imitates sound	6 months		
	Says 2–3 words with meaning	12 months		
7.	**Intellectual development**			
	Begins to repeat actions own body voluntary (hand to mouth) movement permit sucking	4 months		
	Repeat actions that effect an object to get a response	6 months		
	Searches briefly for objects seen being placed elsewhere	6 months		

CHAPTER

17

Psychiatric Nursing: History Taking and Care Plan Format

Name of the student---------------------------------------Course ------------
Date ------------------------ Clinical posting (specialty) ------------------

Demographic Data

Name	Age
Gender	Name of the father/husband name
Education	Occupation
Marital status	Nationality
Language spoken	Religion
Home town/city/address	Income
Date of admission	IP No.
Provisional diagnosis	Treatment received on arrival to hospital
Informant	

History of Present Illness

Ask any or all of the following as appropriate and write summary below

What problem made you to come to hospital	
When this symptoms started	
Any precipitating factors/aggravating (what were you doing at that time)	
Was the onset sudden or gradual	
How often does the problem occur	
Duration of present problem	
Has the problem occurred before	
Did you try home or other remedies to cure the problem	

Contd...

Contd...

Significant area affected	
Reason for admission	
Direct admission	
Referred by others	

Any relevant information ---

Socioeconomic status	Living locality: Urban/rural/semi urban/slum Housing condition: Pucca/kutcha Water supply: Tap/ borewell/ open well Family income : ----------------Rs Occupation: -----------------
Past medical history	History of previous mental illness—yes/no History of previous hospitalization, if yes History of treatment ----------------------- Any medical events: such as head injury, surgery, DM, hypertension, convulsion
Past psychiatric history	Any hospitalization—yes/no Treatment taken—yes/no Psychological therapies ------------------- Previous episode if any in detail-------------------------
Family history	History of major physical illness/psychiatric illness/drug abuse/ alcohol use/ suicid. Genogram --
Personal history	Perinatal history. Antenatal period—eventful/uneventful exposure to radiation/drugs/infection Natal: Birth: premature/normal delivery/ forceps/cesarian section/instrumental delivery. Birth cry: Immediate/delayed Bonding: Immediate/delayed Reaction of parents to child birth------- Postnatal complications: Underweight/infection/ separation from mother/delayed breastfeeding
Childhood history	Parent relationship with the child: Harmonious/ disturbed Developmental mile stone as per age: Normal/delayed Relationship with family members: Normal/disturbed Immunization: Received as per schedule. Yes/no feeding: breast feed/artificial mode Weaning : Response to weaning------------- Behavior: Temper tantrum/thumb sucking/stuttering/ head banging/nail biting/night mares

Contd...

Contd...

Educational history	Academic achievement: Normal/underachiever Extracurricular activity: Normal/underachiever Relationship with teacher: Good/disturbed Attendance to school: Adequate/ frequent absent Relationship with peers: Normal/not adjusting Attitude toward schooling: Positive/negative Reason for discontinuing of study (if any: ---
Play history	Participate in games sports yes/no. Types of game played: Like to play individual/with group Involvement in imaginative play: Yes/no Relationship with playmates: Good/not adjustable
Puberty	Age of menarche--------------------------- Reaction to menarche-------------------- Regularity of cycle----------------------- Duration of flow------------------------
Occupational history	Job started at what age------------------- Relationship with superior/colleagues/subordinates: Satisfactory/not satisfactory Frequent change in job if any ----------------------- Period of unemployment------------------------- Job satisfaction--------------------------------
Sexual and marital history	Type of marriage---------------------- Duration of marriage-------------------- Relationship with spouse-------------------- Responsibilities shared with spouse---------------------- Premarital or extramarital relationship----------------------------- Sexual relationship: Satisfactory/unsatisfactory Marital disharmony if any----------------------------------
Interest and hobbies	Relationship with neighbors---------------- Hobbies------------------------------ Leisure time activities------------------------
Pre-morbid personality	Respect moral value: Yes/no Living pattern: Reality/fantasy Utilizing strength and abilities--------------------------- Social relationship with others----------------------- Type of personality------------------------ Use of leisure time------------------------------- Religious beliefs------------------------------------- Predominant mood: Anxious/pessimistic/optimistic/ stable/fluctuating Personality: Shy/suspicious/irritable/self centered/ impulsive/unconfident/obsessional

- Mental status examination. Refer to mental status examination format
- Refer to neurological examination.

Investigation

Sl. No.	Name of the investigation	Patient value	Normal value	Remarks

Medication

Name of the drugs	Dosage/route/ frequency	Action	Side effect	Nurses responsibilities

Nursing Care Plan

Assessment	Nursing diagnosis	Objectives	Nursing intervention	Rationale	Evaluation

- Health education
- Conclusion
- Reference

Mental Status Examination

History Taking

Identification Data

Name	Age
Sex	Father/spouse
Education	Occupation
Income	Marital status
Religion	IP number
Diagnosis	
Informant	
History of present psychiatric illness (according to patient)	
History of past psychiatric illness (according to patient relatives)	
Past medical history	
Family history	
Personal history	

A general appearance and behavior Body built --	
Level of grooming	Normal/stability dressed/overdressed/ idiosyncratically dressed
Level of cleanliness	Adequate/inadequate/overtly clean
Level of consciousness	Fully conscious and alert/drowsy/stupors/comatose
Mode of entry	Came willingly/persuaded/brought using physical force
Cooperativeness	Normal/more than so/less than so
Eye to eye contact	Maintained/difficult/not maintained
Psychomotor activity	Normal/increased/decreased
Rapport	Spontaneous/difficult/not establish
Gesturing	Grimace /tics/mannerism
Posturing	Normal posture/catatonic posture
Other movement	Stereotype/tremors/extrapyramidal
Other catatonic phenomena	Automatic obedience/ negativism/excessive cooperation/waxy flexibility/echopraxia/echolalia
Conversion and dissociate sign	

Contd...

Contd...

Compulsive acts or rituals	
Hallucinatory behavior	
Speech	
Initiation	Spontaneous/speaks when spoken to/minimal/ mute
Reaction time	Normal/delayed/shortened/difficulty
Rate	Normal /slow/rapid
Productivity	Monosyllabic/elaborate replies/pressured
Volume	Normal/increased/decreased
Tone	Normal variation/monotonous
Relevance	Fully relevance/sometimes off target/irrelevant
Stream	Normal /circumstantial/tangential
Coherence	Fully coherent/loosening of association
Others	Rhyming/echolalia/neologism

Sample of speech (is response to open ended questions)	Q : A :
Mood	Objective: Labile /angry/hopeless/retarded thinking/thought block / muddled or unclear thinking / thinking/flight of ideas

Thought Stream	Normal/formal thought disorder (specify with a sample of speech)
Content Ideas/delusions of	Worthlessness/helplessness/guilt/hypochondrial/ poverty/nihilistic/death wishs/suicidal/grandiose/ reference / control/ persecution/bizarre
Thought alienation phenomena	Thought insertion/thought withdrawal/thought broadcasting
Obsessional/compulsive phenomena	Thoughts/images /ruminations/doubts/impulsive rituals
Perception	
Hallucinations	
Somatic passivity	
Orientation	Time: Normal/impaired Place : Normal/impaired Person: Normal/impaired

Contd...

Contd...

Attention	Normal/impaired
Concentration	Normally sustained/sustained with difficulty/distractible
Memory	Immediate: Intact/absent Recent : Intact/absent Remote : Intact/impaired
Intelligence (performance in studies)	General information
Insight	a. Awareness of abnormal behavior/experience yes/no b. Attribution to physical cause yes/no c. Recognition of personal responsibility. yes/no d. Willingness to take treatment yes/no
Judgment	a. Personal: Intact/impaired b. Social: Intact/impaired c. Reaction to situation: Intact/impaired

General information whereabouts: ---------------------------------------

Performance Evaluation: Assessing the Neurological System

Sl. No.	Performance Criteria	S	U	NP	Comments
	Assessment				
1.	Assessed level of consciousness Assessed eye opening responses				
2.	Eliciting verbal responses • is he alert • is he lethargic or drowsy • is he getting restless • is he irritable				
3.	Elicited motor response. Ask the patient to • Open his eye • Stick out his tongue • Hold up his arms • Squeeze and release finger				
4.	Assessed for motor response **Testing muscle strength** • Muscle tone • Posture • Muscle coordination • Reflexes • Abdominal movement				

Contd...

Contd...

Sl. No.	Performance Criteria	S	U	NP	Comments
	Supported and instruct him to straighten his leg as you apply resistance Evaluate and document client performance incorporate assessment in patient care plan				
5.	**Patellar reflex:** Knee jerk. of a deep tendon reflexes. To elicit this reflex when patients lying down, placed hand under his knee to raise and flex it. Then tap his patellar tendon just below the knee with a reflex hammer. if he expands normally, his leg will extend				
6.	**Plantar reflex:** Stroked the lateral aspect of the sole of the patient's foot. The normal response is flexion of the toes. The babinski response is abnormal. The great toe wills dorsiflex and the other toes fan. This indicates an upper neuron lesion				
7.	Assessed for abnormal movements • Example • Seizures • Tremors • Convulsions				
8.	Assessed for sensory function • Central and peripheral vision (visual acuity and visual fields) • Hearing and ability to understand verbal communication • Superficial sensation (light touch, pain) • Deep sensation like muscle and joint pain or sense of muscle and joint position				
9.	**Danger Signals Noted:** Any of the following conditions in patient s with neurological problems may indicate a serious perhaps life threatening situation • Decreasing level of consciousness • Fixed, dialted pupil • Decorticate or decerebrate movements • Altered pattern of respiration				
	Planning				
1.	Developed individualized goals for assessment				
2.	Identified expected outcomes				
	Implementation				
1.	Mental and emotional status				
2.	Assessed client orientation state				

Contd...

Contd...

Sl. No.	Performance Criteria	S	U	NP	Comments
3.	Asked question about person, place, and time if client initial answers were inappropriate				
4.	Tested response to question				
	Behaviors and appearance				
1.	Observed of client behavior/ mood throughout assessment				
2.	Observed manner of client speech				
	Language function				
1.	Assessed ability of client to understand spoken or written words and to express self				
	Intellectual function				
1.	Assessed clients immediate recall				
2.	Assessed clients recent memory				
3.	Assessed client past memory				
4.	Assessed client knowledge of illness or hospitalization				
5.	Tested clients ability to explain meaning of stated proverb				
6.	Asked client to identify similarity or association between simple terms or concepts				
	Cranial nerve function				
1.	Correctly assessed function of each of twelve cranial nerves				
	Sensory function				
2.	Tested sensory function to pain, temperature, light tough, vibration, position, two point discrimination				
3.	Measured sensation by applying stimuli in random, unpredictable order				
4.	Compared sensation in symmetric body parts				
5.	Asked client to say when particular stimulus perceived				
	Motor function				
1.	Assessed gait, stance, muscle strength, and tone				
2.	Assessed client ability to perform rapid repeating movement of upper extremity				

Contd...

Contd...

Sl. No.	Performance Criteria	S	U	NP	Comments
3.	Assessed clients ability to perform skilled motor act				
4.	Assessed clients upper extremity coordination				
5.	Measured clients ability to perform skilled motor act				
6.	Assessed client ability to perform rapid, repeated movement of lower extremities				
7.	Performed Romberg test				
8.	Asked client to close eyes, stand on one foot, then the other				
	Reflexes				
1.	Assessed deep tendon reflexes correctly and graded according to scale				
	Evaluation				
1.	Compared findings with normal assessment characteristics				
2.	Identified unexpected outcomes				
	Recording and reporting				
1.	Recorded assessment findings in nurses notes				
2.	Reported abnormalities to nurse in charge or physician				

Signature of Student ---------------------------------------

Signature of Clinical Instructor -------------------------------

CHAPTER

18

Midwifery Procedure

Midwifery and Obstetrical Nursing Case Study (selected patient will be pregnancy associated with pregnancy with diabetes, or hypertension, etc.)

Name of the Student---Class --------------------
Date of Case study/Nursing Care Started-----------Date of Completion--------------
Name of the Hospital --

History Taking and Physical Examination

Demographic Data

Name of the Mother	
Age	Husband Age
Date of first visit	Date of booking
Language spoken	Religion
Occupation: Husband Wife	Family income
Education : Husband Wife	Address

Prenatal Record

Gestation at first visit	EDD
LMP	Para/Gravida
Chief complaints	History of urinary tract infection/hypertension/asthma/epilepsy/psychiatry disorders/diabetes/cardiac conditions
Comments	

Obstetric History

Types of family: nuclear/joint/extended	Type of marriage: consanguineous marriage/non consanguineous
Frequency, duration and amount of menstrual flow	No of children Multiple pregnancy.
Marital, relationship satisfactory/nonsatisfactory	Menorrhagia/intermenstural spotting
Dysfunctional uterine bleeding (DUB)	Remarks
Genetic history: cerebral palsy/congenital anomalies/cystic fibrosis/Down syndrome/ hemophilia/mental retardation/muscular dystrophy/neural tube defect/sickle cell disease or trait/ thalassemia B	
LMP	
Calculation of estimated due date (EDD)	
Determination of the present number of weeks of gestation	
Rh and ABO blood type	
Previous pregnancy and delivery	
Place of delivery: Hospital/home	
Length of labor	
Type of delivery	
Spontaneous/instrumental or cesarean section	
Any obstetric, medical problem during pregnancy, labor, or delivery	

Present History

Present pregnancy complaints	
Possible problems in all trimesters of pregnancy	Headache/dizziness/visual disturbance/syncope/ fatigue/nauses/vomiting/heartburn/breast changes/ shortness of breath/abdominal pain/vaginal bleeding/ vaginal discharge/constipation/hemorrhoids
Bowel habits	Regular/irregular
Skin	Abdominal wall/groin/vulva/anal region
Lymphatic system	Enlarged glands/neck axila/groin/lymphangitis

Contd...

Contd...

Vaginal discharge	Red/white
Menstrual history	Age at menrche ---------------regular/irregular, no of days of bleeding: 3days/5days/8 days

Past Medical History

Previous obstetric history	Anemia/neonatal death/neonatal anomaly/gestational diabetes/hyperemesis gravidarum/incompetent cervix/isoimmunization/polyhydramnios/postpartum depression/pregnancy induced hypertension/preterm labor.
Abortion history	Pregnancy loss/--------------------month and year -------------------sex of the birth---male/female. Type of abortion. Spontaneous/induced/abortion:term/preterm/abortion .congenital abnormalities no syphilis.
Causes of abortion	History of medication----------------------- History of immunization-------------------- History of exposure to radiation------------ History of smoking/tobacco---------------- History of chewing--------------------------
Previous type of delivery	Normal/vaginal/forceps/cesarean section, nature of cesarean section: elective/emergency
Gynecological history	Abnormal PAP Any gynecological surgery Infertility
Cardiovascular history have you suffered any disease	Heart disease/rheumatic fever/mitral valve prolapsed/chronic hypertension/varicosities/thrombophlebitis
Respiratory system	Asthma/allergy
Neurological seizures	
Endocrine disorders	Diabetes mellitus/thyroid disorders
Gastrointestinal disorders	
Renal disorders	
Sexually transmitted disease	Gonorrhea/herpes simplex/syphilis
Other infection	Toxoplasmosis/rubella/chicken pox/cytomegalovirus/AIDS/hepatitis
Psychological history	Abuse or neglect-------------------------- Addiction (drug/alcohol/narcotics)
Other infection	Toxoplasmosis/group B streptococcus/rubella/chicken pox/AIDS/hepatitis

Other Examination

Height of the mother----------------	Blood group------------------------ Rh Typing-------------------------- Hb %----------------------------- BT----------------------------------- CT----------------------------------- VDRL----------------------------------- HBsAg----------------------------------- Urine –sugar---------------------albumin------------ Microscope -------------------------
Abdominal examination	Inspection Uterine size------------------------- Shape of the uterus-------------------- Fetal movement --------------------- Skin changes------------------------- Palpation-girth of the abdomen--- Fundal height-----------------fundal-----------palpation --------------------------------lateral palpation --------- --- Pelvic palpation---------------------------- 1st pelvic grip------------------------------- 2nd pelvic grip ------------------------ Auscultation FHR -------------------right side------- rate/min Rhythm Location------position------------------ Left side-------rate/min Rhythm Location –position
P.V Examination	Cervix------------------------------- Internal os-------------------------------- External os----------------------------- Dilation---------------------------------- Effacement----------------------------- Position--------------------------------------- Presentation------------------------------ Presenting part-------------------------- Adequacy of pelvis------------------------ Discharge-----------------------------

Apgar Scoring

	Sign	0	Neonate score 1 min 5 min	1	Neonate score 1 min 5 min	2	Neonate's score 1 min 5 min
1	Respiratory effort	Absent		Slow, irregular, weak cry		Strong cry	
2	Heart rate	Absent		Slow, less than 100		Over 100	
3	Muscle tone	Limp		Some flexion of limb		Active movement	
4	Reflex response to flicking of foot	Absent		Facial grimace		Cry	
5	Color	Blue pale		Body pink, limbs blue		Completely pink	

0-2 severe asphyxia
3-4 moderate asphyxia
5-7 no asphyxia
Still born/macerated -----------------------causes ------------------------------------
Treatment at birth ---
Birth injuries --
Congenital abnormalities------------------------
Medication given --
Significant investigation if present
Significant medication--
Type of diet ---

Comparative Study According to Text and Patient

Disease as per text	Disease as per patient
Related anatomy and physiology	
Etiology	
Risk factors	
Clinical manifestation	
Pathophysiology	
Assessment and diagnosis findings	
Medical management	
Nursing management	
Evaluation	

Summary
References

Investigation Done

Date	Name of investigation	Normal value	Patient value	Significant result

Medical diagnosis ....

Drug Management

Name of the drug	Dosage and frequency	Route	Action	Side effect	Nursing investigation

List of Nursing Diagnosis

1. ....
2. ....
3. ....

Nursing Care Plan

Nursing assessment	Nursing diagnosis	Objectives	Nursing intervention	Evaluation

Performance Evaluation of Midwifery Nursing Procedures

Performance Evaluation: Antenatal Abdominal Examination

An abdominal examination is carried out to gain information about fetal growth and well-being. The findings from an abdominal examination change throughout the pregnancy.

1. In early pregnancy fundus cannot be palpable per abdomen.
2. From about 12 weeks it is palpable just above the symphysis pubis.
3. At the 16th week it is halfway between the symphysis pubis and the umbilicus.
4. By 24 weeks the fundus is palpable at the umbilicus and fetal heart sounds can be heard with Pinards stethoscope.
5. At 30 weeks the fundus can be felt midway between the umbilicus and the xiphisternum.
6. By 36 weeks the fundus will have reached the xiphisternum.
7. By 38 weeks the mother may experience 'lightening', (more room at the top of the fundus as the presenting part sinks into the pelvis).

Purpose

To describe the method by which an antenatal abdominal examination should be:

Procedure

Sl. No.	Performance Criteria	S	U	NP	Comments
	Assessment				
1.	Collected and prepared the equipment				
2.	Explained the procedure to the woman				
3.	Asked the woman to empty her bladder just prior to the procedure				

Contd...

Contd...

Sl. No.	Performance Criteria	S	U	NP	Comments
4.	Asked the woman to lie as flat as possible, with just a pillow under her head				
	Implementation				
1.	Washed and dried hands				
2.	Drawn the curtains around the bed and exposed only the woman's abdomen				
3.	Observed for any scars or striae gravindarum ('stretch marks')				
4.	Placed one hand on the fundus and estimated fundal size (Fundal size can also be measured by using a tape measure stretched from the fundus to the symphysis pubis with one centimeter equaling approximately one week)				
5.	Palpated the abdomen at the fundus to determine presenting part				
6.	Palpated laterally to locate the fetal back .One hand is used to palpate along one side of the abdomen				
7.	Determined the nature of the presenting part by performing a gentle pelvic palpation. Placed one hand on either side of the uterus near the pelvic brim				
8.	Auscultated the fetal heart by using the chosen method on the side of the abdomen on which the back felt				
9.	Explained the findings to the mother and answer her questions (if any)				
10.	Assisted the mother from the couch/bed				
11.	Washed and dried hands				
	Recording and reporting				
12.	Documented the findings appropriately. Reported to sister incharge				

Note: The size of the abdomen should correspond with the expected gestational age. If there is any discrepancy, the LMP should be checked. If there are continuing concerns the mother should be referred to a doctor and for an ultrasound scan.

Signature of Student --

Signature of Clinical Instructor ---

Performance Evaluation: Abortion Care of—Missed

Definition

Missed abortion usually present following threatened abortion.

It is diagnosed by ultrasound, bleeding occurs between the gestation sac and the uterine wall and the embryo dies, forming blood clots. It is also known as carneous mole. The uterus does not increase in size and signs of pregnancy will disappear. The women may present with slight bleeding or a brownish discharge.

Purpose

1. To provide support and guidance to the woman and the family.
2. To relieve the woman's discomfort.
3. To carry out treatment prescribed.

Procedure

Sl. No.	Performance Criteria	S	U	NP	Comments
	Assessment				
1.	Admitted to the Antenatal/Gynae ward and made patient as comfortable as possible				
	Implementation				
1.	Observed and examined the bleeding per vagina				
2.	Recorded vital signs as appropriate				
3.	Explained all procedures to the women				
4.	Prepared the woman for ultrasound as per the requirement				
5.	Followed ultrasound for the confirmation of missed abortion				
6.	Managed the case as per doctor's order (for evacuation of retained products of conception/ prostaglandin's according to gestation)				
7.	Supported the woman and answered her queries				
8.	Explained all procedures to the women				
9.	Continued care as per preoperative and postoperative procedures				
10.	Following surgery observed bleeding per vagina				
11.	Given psychological support to the women				

Contd...

Contd...

Sl. No.	Performance Criteria	S	U	NP	Comments
	Recording and reporting				
1.	Given follow up appointment as directed				
2.	Documented appropriately				
3.	Informed pertinent information to ward incharge nurse				

Signature of Student --

Signature of Clinical Instructor --------------------------------

Performance Evaluation: Abortion Care of—Threatened

Definition

Threatened abortion is slight bleeding usually during the first trimester. It may be painless or associated with slight lower abdominal pain or backache.

Heavy or increased bleeding may proceed to inevitable abortion, this can be a complete or incomplete abortion.

Purpose

1. To provide support and guidance to women.
2. To carry out treatment as prescribed.

Procedure

Sl. No.	Performance Criteria	S	U	NP	Comments
	Assessment				
1.	Admitted to the antenatal/Gynae ward and make as comfortable as possible				
2.	Advised the women to maintain bed rest until 24 hrs after the bleeding has ceased				
3.	Observed the bleeding per vagina				
4.	Recorded vital signs 4 hourly				
5.	Checked the women blood group				
6.	Mild sedative given as per doctor order				
7.	Prepared the woman for ultrasound				
8.	Supported the woman and answer her questions				

Contd...

Contd...

Sl. No.	Performance Criteria	S	U	NP	Comments
9.	Performed vulval swabbing twice daily, to minimize discomfort for the women, as long as the discharge persist				
10.	Assisted the Doctor to perform a Speculum examination between 24 to 48 hrs after the bleeding has stopped				
11.	Encouraged the women to commence gentle ambulation 24 hours after the bleeding has stopped				
12.	Given advice on the importance of rest on her return home				
13.	Encouraged women in case of future pregnancy early booking				
14.	On discharge advise the woman to attend her nearest parent institution for antenatal booking				
	Recorded and reporting				
1.	Informed doctor on her condition				
2.	Reported to charge nurse, about the care provided				

Signature of Student --

Signature of Clinical Instructor --------------------------------

Performance Evaluation: Antepartum Hemorrhage Care of

Definition

Antepartum hemorrhage is defined as bleeding from the genital tract after the 24th week of pregnancy and before the birth of the baby.

APH is a serious condition, which may result in the death of the mother or the baby.

Types

1. **Placenta previa** which is painless bleeding from separation of an abnormally sited placenta.
2. **Abruptio placenta** which is bleeding from separation of a normally situated placenta.
3. **Extra placental bleeding** is incidental or associated bleeding which sometime occurs from some other part of the birth canal, e.g. cervical polyp.

Note

The order of the observations will depend on the condition of the women. A vaginal examination should not be performed.

Procedure

Sl. No.	Performance Criteria	S	U	NP	Comments
	Assessment				
1.	Informed obstetrician when APH is diagnosed				
2.	Obtained a history of the events from the mother and/or attendant				
	Implementation				
1.	Explained any procedure to the woman				
2.	Observed the mother for pallor or breathlessness				
3.	Recorded vital signs				
4.	Observed the blood loss and ascertain how much has been lost prior to admission				
5.	Observed the abdomen and perform a gentle examination				
6.	Auscultated the fetal heart and ask if there are fetal movements				
7.	Taken blood for hemoglobin estimation, blood count coagulation factor, specimen for cross matching and any other investigation as ordered by the doctor. This can be done when inserting canula				
8.	Cross matched 2 units of blood				
9.	Commence an intravenous line with Hartman's solution				
10.	Maintained bed rest until the bleeding ceases and provide bathroom facilities only when bleeding ceases				
11.	Performed a cardiotocograph				
12.	Admitted or transfer to the appropriate ward/ department				
	Ongoing care				
13.	Performed vulval toilet regularly while there is bleeding				
14.	Assisted the doctor to perform a speculum examination after the bleeding has stopped				

Contd...

Contd...

Sl. No.	Performance Criteria	S	U	NP	Comments
15.	Prepared the mother for ultrasound				
16.	Documented and record findings as appropriate				
17.	Noted the mother's blood group				
18.	The following observation done which will assist in arriving at a provisional diagnosis – Pain, onset of bleeding, amount of visible blood loss, degree of shock, tenderness of the abdomen, lie, presentation, engagement, and audibility of the fetal heart.				
	Recording and reporting				
1.	Recorded procedure in nurses notes				
2.	Reported to charge nurse, about the care provided				

Signature of Student --------------------------------------

Signature of Clinical Instructor ------------------------------

Performance Evaluation: Cervical Cerclage: Preparation for Surgery

Definition

Cervical cerclage is a surgical procedure in which a suture is used to close the cervix during pregnancy to prevent miscarriage.

Purpose

To treat cervical incompetence during pregnancy, in order to prevent miscarriage. It is usually done between 14 to 16 weeks of pregnancy.

Procedure

The procedure must be explained to the women by the doctor on admission and consent obtained. The nurse preparing the women ensures that the women has a clear understanding of the procedure and explains the nursing preparation.

Sl. No.	Performance Criteria	S	U	NP	Comments
	Assessment				
1.	Kept the woman fasting overnight				
2.	Ensured that the woman is wearing an identification bracelet with correct personal information				

Contd...

Contd...

Sl. No.	Performance Criteria	S	U	NP	Comments
3.	Assessed the preoperative information received by the women is complete and understood properly				
4.	Instructed the women to have shower on the morning of operation				
	Implementation				
1.	Checked that the women has undergone relevant preoperative investigations, e.g. X-ray, ECG, pelvic scan, blood tests, urine tests and that these results are in woman's notes				
2.	Recorded the women pulse, blood pressure, respiration, temperature and weight (if appropriate)				
3.	Ensured that the woman empties her bladder before premedication is given				
4.	Completed preoperative check list with the related information. a. Checked when woman last had food or drink (if she has eaten recently the anesthetist must be informed) b. Ensured the prosthesis, dentures and contact lenses are removed and confirmed that woman has no loose teeth c. Removed all jewelery, cosmetics, nail polish etc. d. Given theater dress				
5.	Valuables placed in the hospital custody and recorded as per hospital policy				
6.	Checked the consent form is correctly completed, signed and dated				
7.	Checked that the woman has undergone preanesthetic assessment by the anesthetist				
8.	Given premedication, as prescribed according to the order, to reduce anxiety				
9.	Advised the woman to remain in bed to prevent injury due to the effect of premedication				
10.	Ensured that the women can reach the call bell and instructed her to use it if she needs the nurse				
11.	Documented preoperative preparation, premedication given with time and date				
12.	Ensured that all relevant investigations reports are sent to theater along with woman				
13.	Handed over the patient to theater nurse with proper documents				

Contd...

Contd...

Sl. No.	Performance Criteria	S	U	NP	Comments
14.	Informed relatives time of arrival, condition of patient after surgery				

Signature of Student ---------------------------------------

Signature of Clinical Instructor -------------------------------

Performance Evaluation: Antenatal Examination at First Visit

Definition

Initial GENERAL and ABDOMINAL assessment performed when a pregnant woman attends the antenatal clinic for the first time. A complete health history is obtained before the procedure is carried out.

The examination is usually done by a specialist obstetrician or a medical officer. If no medical doctor is available in a remote Health Center a registered midwife or nurse can do the examination and refer any medical or obstetric problem to a doctor at the appropriate Regional Referral or Tertiary Hospital for investigation and management.

Procedure

Sl. No.	Performance Criteria	S	U	NP	Comments
	Assessment				
1.	Received the woman, with smile and asked her name and introduced self by name and job title. Asked about her and family health				
2.	Asked her to collect midstream specimen of urine. Tested the urine for protein, sugar and ketones and send the rest to the laboratory for asymptomatic bacterial screening				
	Implementation				
1.	Measured height and weight without footwear				
2.	Obtained baseline information for monitoring alert like > 80 kg obesity risk < 40 kg malnutrition and small pelvis risks				
3.	Measured blood pressure, ensured using correct method by using correct cuff and reading of 140/90 (more may indicate PIH. Rechecking is necessary after 20–30 minutes in case of variation)				

Physical Examination

1.	Provided privacy. Kept doors/curtains closed				
2.	Checked hair for color and head for lice and dandruff				
3.	**The face:** Observed facial expression for signs of anxiety, depression, pallor, pigmentation and edema (after 28 weeks)				
4.	Checked conjunctiva for degree of redness				
5.	Examined mouth for condition of gums and teeth				
6.	**The neck:** Palpated below posterior angle of the jaw bones for swollen nodes				
7.	Palpated lobes of the thyroid glands on both sides of the trachea just below the cricoid cartilage (Adam's apple)				
8.	Turned the head to the side and observed the carotid vein				
9.	Reviewed medical histories, for specific conditions indicated by observations, and also ascertain history by checking with woman				
10.	**Chest and Lungs:** Assisted woman with necessary position, to hear the heart and lung sounds				
11.	**The breasts:** Explained the reason for examining her breasts				
12.	Exposed both breasts fully				
13.	Inspected for symmetry of size, shape and appearance of skin				
14.	Palpated for lumps and nodules				
15.	Palpated from the auxillary tail then the breast in decreasing circles at point, to find out any irregularities/tenderness				
16.	Gently squeezed nipple to note color and type of secretion				
17.	Showed professional concern and sensitiveness throughout the procedure				
18.	Discussed normal changes as needed				
19.	Given education required for antenatal preparation of lactation. Encouraged her to wear a supportive bra				
20.	Referred abnormal finding to the sister incharge promptly				
21.	Noted color of palms and nail beds				
22.	Examined the legs, ankles and feet for: shape and equal length				
23.	Advised to keep the feet elevated when seated to reduce edema and to Increase the rest periods, lying on her left side to improve renal flow and excretion of fluid				
24.	Advised avoid extra salt to food and restrict intake of salty foods				

Contd...

Contd...

25.	Advised to increase intake of protein and reduce carbohydrates. Drink at least 6 to 8 glasses of fluid/day to help natural diuresis. Taught to recognize the signs of preeclampsia. And to visit to obstetrician promptly				
26.	Assessed for any varicosities and it causes any pain, any pitting edema and stasis				
27.	Advised to avoid crossing legs at the knees, also to get up and move around every hour if sitting for long periods.				
28.	Taught the woman about the danger signs of condition that put herself and fetus at risk				
29.	Ensured she understood all the instructions.				
	Recording and reporting				
1.	Documented all findings in nurses notes				
2.	Informed sister incharge pertinent information				

Signature of Student ---------------------------------------

Signature of Clinical Instructor -------------------------------

Performance Evaluation: Antenatal Examination First Fetal Movement Recording of

Definition

The counting of fetal movements by the pregnant woman from 28 weeks of gestation is recommended as a simple method for assessing fetal well being. There are two popular methods. One method recommends that the woman sits for a specified period of time up to three times a day and counts total movements. The alternative to this policy is adapted from the 'Cardiff count to Ten' method. Both are discussed below:

Purpose

1. To state the procedure for teaching the counting of fetal movements to pregnant women.
2. To state the correct procedure for filling in the fetal movement chart.
3. To explain the procedure to be followed when the pregnant woman does not feel sufficient fetal movements.

Note: The procedure for counting fetal movements using the 'Three times a day' method and the 'Cardiff count to ten' method has certain common steps. These are steps 1 to 5 below. After this the methods involve different care actions.

Procedure

Sl. No.	Performance Criteria	S	U	NP	Comments
	Assessment				
1.	Explained to mother the benefits of counting fetal movements by 28 weeks gestation				
2.	Documented that she has discussed this with the mother and signs and dates the antenatal card				
3.	Checked the fetal movement chart at visit or daily and reinforces the women the importance of counting fetal movements				
4.	Documented her discussion about fetal movements at every antenatal visit				
5.	Given a chart to the mother in the language she understands and has an explanation in her own language				

Recording Fetal Movements Using the 'three times a day' Method

First follow steps 1 to 5 outlined overleaf then continue with steps 6 to 11 below:

6.	The mother is advised to count fetal movements for three one hour periods every day over a 12 hour period				
7.	The mother advised to tick on the chart every time she feel a movements and stop after one hour				
8.	The mother is advised to choose times when she is able to concentrate on fetal movement counting (e.g. after other children have gone to school or when the family are resting after lunch)				
9.	The mother is informed that if she has not felt at least ten movements by the end of the third counting session she should inform her gynecologist				
10.	The mother is advised to attend hospital for a CTG if has not felt sufficient movements				
11.	The fetal movement chart, stored carefully in the obstetric notes after the pregnancy is finished				

Counting Fetal Movements Using the 'Cardiff count to ten' Method

First follow steps 1 to 5 on the first page then continue with steps 12 to 16 outlined below:

12.	The mother is advised to start counting fetal movements at the same time every day				
13.	The mother should tick on the chart every time she feel a movement and then stop when she gets to ten or when the eight hour period is completed				

Contd...

Contd...

14.	The mother should write down the time each day when she has felt the tenth movement (If mother is unable to write then advise her to relate the tenth movement to a daily event)				
15.	The mother is informed that if she has not felt the tenth movement by the end of the twelve hour period she should telephone to her gynecologist or visit to the nearest hospital or health center				
16.	The fetal movement chart should be stored carefully in the obstetric notes when the pregnancy is finished				

Signature of Student ---------------------------------------

Signature of Clinical Instructor -------------------------------

Performance Evaluation: Oral Glucose Challenge Test (OGCT)

Definition

A routine screening test performed during pregnancy to determine the blood glucose levels are within normal limits.

Purpose

1. To determine blood glucose levels.
2. To exclude gestational diabetes.

Procedure

Sl. No.	Performance Criteria	S	U	NP	Comments
	Assessment				
1.	Identified the woman who requires OGCT				
2.	Explained the procedure to the women				
3.	Obtained information from women and completed appropriate forms				
4.	Washed and dried hands (refer to hand washing procedure)				
5.	Blood is taken by the appropriate personnel and put it into the appropriate blood tube (refer to venipuncture procedure)				
6.	Ensured that blood tube is labeled with the relevant women details				
7.	Dissolved glucose in 200–300 mL water				
8.	Given glucose solution to women and asked her to drink at once				

Contd...

Contd...

Sl. No.	Performance Criteria	S	U	NP	Comments
9.	Noted the time that the glucose solution was given				
10.	After one hour, taken the blood sample and put it into the appropriate blood tube				
11.	Ensured that the blood tube is labeled with the relevant women details				
12.	Followed hospital procedure for the collection and transportation of specimens to the laboratory				
13.	Documented appropriately				

Signature of Student ---

Signature of Clinical Instructor ------------------------------

Performance Evaluation: Glucose Tolerance Test (GTT)

Definition

Glucose tolerance test is a screening test, to determine the postprandial blood glucose level.

Purpose

1. To determine blood glucose levels.
2. To exclude diabetes mellitus.

Procedure

Sl. No.	Performance Criteria	S	U	NP	Comments
	Assessment				
1.	Identified woman				
2.	Explained the procedure to the woman				
3.	Ensured that the woman is fasting and has had carbohydrate diet for three days prior to test				
4.	Obtained information from women and completed appropriate forms				
5.	Washed and dried hands				
6.	Blood is taken by appropriate personnel and collected in the appropriate tube				
7.	Ensured that the blood tube is labeled with the relevant women details				
8.	Dissolved glucose in 200–300 mL water				

Contd...

Contd...

Sl. No.	Performance Criteria	S	U	NP	Comments
9.	Given glucose solution to the women and asked her to drink completely at a time				
10.	Noted the time that the glucose solution was given				
11.	After two hours, taken a blood sample and collected in the appropriate blood tube				
12.	Ensured that the blood tube is labeled with the relevant women details				
13.	Followed hospital procedure for the collection and transportation of specimens to the laboratory				
14.	Documented appropriately				
15.	Provided food and drink as required by the women				

Signature of Student ---------------------------------------

Signature of Clinical Instructor ------------------------------

Performance Evaluation: History Taking—the Antenatal

Booking Interview

Definition

The antenatal booking is an assessment of the physical, social, psychological and emotional state of the pregnant woman.

Purpose

1. To obtain the medical, obstetric and family history.
2. To arrange suitable antenatal care for the pregnancy.
3. To book confinement in a setting with appropriate facilities and professional expertise.
4. To stress the importance of antenatal care and the Maternal Health Card.
5. To give advice about nutrition during pregnancy and other health matters.
6. To discuss and advise on breastfeeding.
7. To discuss and plan individualized care and birth plans.

If using an appointment system, allow adequate time for each interview, health education topics and answer woman questions

Equipment

1. Room with comfortable chairs, relaxing atmosphere and privacy. (Refreshments if possible)
2. Address card and tetanus toxoid card.

3. Teaching aids, charts, etc.
4. Leaflets about antenatal care, breastfeeding, nutrition, etc.
5. A nurse/mid wife with good communication skills and who speaks the appropriate language.

When to Book

As early as 6 weeks after her last menstrual period her pregnancy has been confirmed by Gravindex test or by ultrasonography.

Early booking provides an early opportunity to improve the nutritional status of the mother, correct her anaemia and educate her about her pregnancy and child birth

How to Book

The woman's details should be written in the Antenatal register/date base, which provides the health institution with essential particulars.

The booking interview should focus on the woman and not be looked upon as a form –filling exercise.

The information should be elicited from the woman in such a way that she does not feel that she is being interrogated.

Questions should be phrased in a way that given the woman the opportunity to speak freely, to improve development of conversation avoids asking questions that will give only yes/no answers.

Procedure

Sl. No.	Performance Criteria	S	U	NP	Comments
	Assessment				
1.	Welcomed the woman using her name and ask about her general well-being				
2.	Introduced self by name and job title				
3.	Ensured privacy whilst obtaining relevant details				
4.	Allowed only one woman at a time in the room				
5.	Filled the woman's name, address and details clearly in the form				
6.	Taken the woman's history carefully and recorded on the relevant section of the maternal health card				
7.	Explained to woman the importance of collecting and recording information relevance to her pregnancy				
8.	During history taking fully utilized, opportunities for health education, e.g. nutrition, diet, breastfeeding etc.				
9.	Checked the woman's tetanus toxoid status (immunized her as required)				

Contd...

Contd...

Sl. No.	Performance Criteria	S	U	NP	Comments
10.	Explained on blood test at different times during her pregnancy, as per the need.				
11.	Explained about head to toe examination, for confirming her health status				
12.	Given the woman opportunity to ask questions throughout the examination				
13.	Upon completion of the booking interview the woman is given an appointment for the next visit and reminded of the importance of antenatal visit				

Signature of Student ---------------------------------------

Signature of Clinical Instructor -------------------------------

Performance Evaluation: Non Stress Test (NST)

Definition

A non stress test is the monitoring of the fetal heart rate patterns of the fetus in response to fetal movements.

The technique is carried out via external CTG (cardiotocography) monitoring without any stress or stimuli to the fetus.

Purpose

To identify the fetus at risk, of death and morbidity due to intrapartum asphyxia.

Equipment Required

1. CTG monitor with external cardiotocography and tocography transducers and necessary accessories
2. Ultrasound coupling gel
3. Paper towel
4. Remote event marker (optional)
5. Pen for manual marking of fetal movements

Procedure

Sl. No.	Performance Criteria	S	U	NP	Comments
	Assessment				
1.	Checked physicians' order				
2.	Identified the woman				
3.	Explained the procedure to the woman and ensured privacy				

Contd...

Contd...

Sl. No.	Performance Criteria	S	U	NP	Comments
4.	Washed and dried hands				
5.	Allowed the woman to empty her bladder before the procedure				
6.	Carried out routine steps for applying a CTG monitor				
7.	Given woman call bell. Inserted remote event marker into monitor (if available)				
8.	Observed fetal movements by placing a hand on the uterus and marked on the graph paper for each movement, by pressing the appropriate button				
9.	Performed monitoring for 20 minutes unless otherwise indicated				
10.	Continued monitoring and informed the obstetrician a abnormal findings are apparent or tracings are inaccurate				
11.	When CTG monitoring is completed, allowed the woman to mobilize but asked her not to leave until the CTG has been reviewed				
12.	Had tracing reviewed and signed by the obstetrician				
13.	Advised woman on all follow up appointments and the importance of keeping these appointments				
14.	Ensured that the CTG tracing has been labeled correctly and that it is filed appropriately				
15.	Documented appropriately				

Signature of Student ---------------------------------------

Signature of Clinical Instructor ------------------------------

Performance Evaluation: Ultrasound Preparation For

Definition

Ultrasound is the use of reflected high sound waves as they travel in tissue to produce a picture on a screen which is used to diagnose the presence, size and position of a mass.

Purpose

1. To confirm and diagnose pregnancy.
2. To accurately assess gestational age in early pregnancy.
3. To detect a dead fetus.

4. To diagnose extra uterine pregnancy
5. To detect a pelvic mass, cyst, fibroid or retained products of conception
6. To check the fetus for abnormality
7. To localize the placenta
8. Diagnosis in molar pregnancy
9. To detect the presence of retro placental clots in Abruptio Placenta
10. To determine fetal well-being as part of a biophysical profile
11. To observe fetal movements
12. To determine fetal presentation
13. To estimate fetal weight
14. To estimate liquor volume and obtain amniotic fluid index
15. Serial scans can aid in the diagnosis of IUGR
16. To undertake Doppler to estimate umbilical cord blood flow

Equipment

1. Ultrasound machine
2. Ultrasound coupling gel
3. Appropriate transducers
4. Tissue paper
5. Polaroid film

Procedure

Sl. No.	Performance Criteria	S	U	NP	Comments
	Assessment				
1.	**PREPARATION PHASE** Arranged ultrasound appointment as appropriate				
2.	Given instructions to the woman regarding preparation for ultrasound and the location of the department where the ultrasound is to be performed				
3.	As full bladder is required given the woman 1 liter of water an hour of the ultrasound				
4.	Ensured ultrasound is performed as soon as possible after the woman's bladder is full				
5.	**PROCEDURE** Verified the doctor's order				
6.	Identified the woman				
7.	Explained the procedure to the woman/husband				
8.	Ensured privacy				
9.	Washed and dried hands				
10.	Collected and prepared the equipment				

Contd...

Contd...

Sl. No.	Performance Criteria	S	U	NP	Comments
11.	Ensured the woman has a full bladder				
12.	Positioned the woman on an examination couch so that she can see the ultrasound screen (if she wishes)				
13.	Ensured comfort of the woman throughout the procedure				
14.	Covered the woman allowing only the abdomen to be exposed				
15.	Protected the woman's clothes/underwear from gel by tucking paper towels into her underwear				
16.	Allowed for a relaxed and informative atmosphere during the procedure				
17.	Prepared to assist the obstetrician during the procedure				
18.	Referred all questions to the obstetrician				
19.	Wiped gel from the abdomen and covered the woman as soon as the procedure is over				
20.	Asked the obstetrician to speak to the expectant parents as soon as possible				
21.	Directed the woman to the toilet immediately on completion of the ultrasound (if she has a full bladder)				
22.	Ensured that the woman has all her follow up appointments				
23.	Documented appropriately				

Signature of Students ---------------------------------------

Signature of Clinical Instructor ------------------------------

Performance Evaluation: Admission—Mother and Baby to the Postnatal Ward

To ensure correct observation and identification of the postnatal mother and her baby.

Procedure

Sl. No.	Performance Criteria	S	U	NP	Comments
	Assessment				
1.	Received the mother by wheelchair (trolley) with her baby to the postnatal ward				

Contd...

Contd...

Sl. No.	Performance Criteria	S	U	NP	Comments
2.	Placed the mother in an appropriately prepared bed and the baby in a cradle next to her				
3.	Checked the mother' ID band (Two nurses examine the baby to confirm the sex and the presence of 2 name bands)				
4.	Received the reports from delivery room nurse about relevant details of the mother history, labor and delivery and her condition since delivery				
5.	Received reports of baby such as sex, weight, apgar score, urine and meconium has been passed, medication given and condition of the baby, and Breastfeeding has been initiated etc.				
6.	All documents are collected from the labor room staff as per hospital policy				
7.	Both nurses checked the Child Health Card and Birth Notification form				
8.	The ward nurse examined the mother to ascertain her condition upon transfer by: • Palpating the uterus • Examining the lochia • Ensuring the bladder is empty				
9.	Recorded vital signs				
10.	The baby is examined for skin color, respiration, and condition of the cord				
11.	The baby temperature is checked per axilla				
12.	Ensured the mother is comfortable and offered her a snack/drink				
13.	Completed the relevant chart and placed at the bedside near the mother and baby				
14.	Documented and recorded findings appropriately				

Signature of Student---

Signature of Clinical Instructor ------------------------------

Performance Evaluation: Breast Milk Expression of

Definition

Expression of milk from breasts, is a method of expelling milk from a lactating mother which can be done manually or mechanically by using a breast pump.

Purpose

1. To collect milk for a baby who is unable to suck, i.e. sick.

2. To stimulate lactation incase of baby sick and unable to suck.
3. To relieve engorgement.

Procedure

Sl. No.	Performance Criteria	S	U	NP	Comments
	Assessment				
1.	Identified the mother				
2.	Explained the procedure to the mother				
3.	Ensured privacy				
4.	Washed and dried hands (both nurse and mother)				
5.	Exposed the breast to be expressed				
6.	Cleaned the breasts to remove dried colostrums. (Use of warm compress improves flow of milk)				
7.	Showed the mother to expel the milk by supporting the breast in one hand and gently squeezing the areola between thumb and first finger of other hand. Used sterile container to collect the expelled milk				
8.	Explained the mother the method of using hand pump and electric pump (If mother is expressing milk for baby on a regular basis a hand pump or electric breast pump may be the best to use)				
9.	Helped the mother to wipe the nipple and areola with damp tissue and dry thoroughly, after procedure				
10.	Applied breast pads and well fitting brassiere (if available)				
11.	Stored the milk in fridge (if required) for feed for maximum of 24 hours				
12.	Cleaned and sterilized the equipment and stored appropriately				
13.	Documented appropriately and reported abnormal findings to charge nurse				

Signature of Student---

Signature of Clinical Instructor -------------------------------

Performance Evaluation: Discharge Advice for Mother and Baby

Purpose

The mother should feel confident in her ability to cope with herself and the baby.

Equipment

1. Relevant leaflets as appropriate
2. Contact telephone numbers

Procedure

Sl. No.	Performance Criteria	S	U	NP	Comments
	Assessment				
1.	Mother is given Health Education on normal Lochia, color, consistency, amount, odor and duration of flow				
2.	Reinforced the importance of perineal hygiene and frequent changing of perineal pads				
3.	Instructed on postnatal exercises				
4.	Encouraged on breastfeeding with positive reinforcement and to contact community support group as per hospital policy				
5.	Advised on a well balanced diet including adequate fluids and fiber				
6.	Reinforced initial birth spacing advice				
7.	Prepared all discharge papers, medication and follow up appointments for mother and baby				
8.	Checked the ID bands of mother and baby				
9.	Handed over all information and medication after explanation to mother when relatives arrive				
10.	Documented appropriately				

Signature of Student---

Signature of Clinical Instructor ------------------------------

Performance Evaluation: Perineal Care Postnatal

Definition

Perineal care is an important part of postnatal care. The midwife/nurse should assess the mother's perineum on arrival to the postnatal ward and advise the mother in maintaining perineal hygiene thereafter. Some mothers will need minimal advice and instruction other will need frequent advice and reminding. All women should receive individualized advice according to their needs N.B. Perineal 'routines' e.g. cleaning the perineum with antiseptic solution in the postnatal period is unnecessary and harmful.

Purpose

1. To promote optimum healing of the perineum in the postnatal period.
2. To advise mother on perineal hygiene after childbirth.

Procedure

Sl. No.	Performance Criteria	S	U	NP	Comments
	Assessment				
1.	Explained the procedure to the woman				
2.	Collected equipment, washed hands and put on clean gloves				
3.	Dragged the screens/curtains around the bed				
4.	Informed the woman to remove her trousers and underwear (or raise her nightdress to above the level of her buttocks)				
5.	Informed the woman to dispose of her soiled pad in a yellow disposable bag. Noted quantity and odor of Lochia before disposal				
6.	Instructed the woman to adopt a side lying position				
7.	Noted the condition of the perineum including any grazes, bruising, hemorrhoids, tears or sutures				
8.	Accompanied the woman to the bathroom and explained cleaning of the perineum from front to back with clean warm water. Instructed her to gently pat the perineum dry with toilet tissue				
9.	Advised the woman that an increase in Lochia is normal during/after breastfeeding				
10.	Provided a clean pad. Instructed the woman to wash and dry the perineum and change the pad in the same way after each visit to the toilet to pass urine/have bowels opened				
11.	Advised the woman to report if she feels any discomfort				
12.	Removed gloves, disposed off the soiled equipment correctly and washed hands				
13.	Documented appropriately				

Signature of Student--

Signature of Clinical Instructor -----------------------------

Performance Evaluation: Postnatal Routine Care of the Mother

Definition

Routine daily postnatal observations

Purpose

1. To observe the general condition of the mother, noting her physical and emotional well-being.
2. To identify potential problems in the mother.
3. To enable the mother to become confident in the care of her baby.

Note: Rooming in, is practiced to encourage bonding of the mother and baby

Procedure

Sl. No.	Performance Criteria	S	U	NP	Comments
	Assessment				
1.	Greeted the mother and asked about her feeling. Ensured some privacy by drawing the curtains around the bed				
2.	Washed and dried hands				
3.	Checked temp, pulse and blood pressure				
4.	Examined the breasts and nipples				
5.	Palpated the uterus				
6.	Observed the discharge (lochia), noting the amount, color and odor				
7.	Assessed the mother for any after pains (gave analgesia If required as per the doctors order)				
8.	Checked the mother for emptying bladder and bowel				
9.	Checked the perineum (if episiotomy suture is present care should be taken)				
10.	Checked the legs and noted any swelling				
11.	Encouraged ambulation to rule out DVT, pain or inflammation				
12.	Encouraged the mother to have adequate rest and sleep				
13.	Observed that she is eating well and drinking adequate fluids				
14.	Given health education on Following topics: • Breastfeeding • Nutrition • Immunization • Birth spacing • Hygiene and prevention of infection • Attendance at postnatal clinic				
15.	Documented appropriately				

Signature of Student---

Signature of Clinical Instructor --------------------------------

Performance Evaluation: Bathing a Baby

Definition

Washing a newborn from head to foot to maintain hygiene

Purpose

To clean the baby and to promote comfort.

Note: The role of the Midwife is to first demonstrate the procedure to the Mother and thereafter to supervise and teach the Mother until she is confident.

Procedure

Sl. No.	Performance Criteria	S	U	NP	Comments
	Assessment				
1.	Explained the procedure to the mother				
2.	Encouraged the mother to observe/participate in the procedure				
3.	Assemble all the item required				
4.	Washed hands				
5.	Prepared bath water by checking the temperature				
6.	Checked the baby's temperature per Axilla				
7.	Checked presence of identity bands				
8.	Wrapped and held the baby leaving the head free				
9.	Changed the water at this stage (if necessary)				
10.	Unwrapped the baby in the cot and removed nappy				
11.	Applied soap to hands and washed baby's arms, trunk and legs ensuring that all skin folds and creases are taken care. Then soap the back and buttocks. Rinse and dried hands				
12.	Held the baby firmly but gently using the left arm to support the shoulder, head and neck				
13.	Placed the baby in the bath and rinse the soap off				
14.	Removed the baby from the bath and laid on the towel. Dried all over ensuring skin folds are thoroughly dried				
15.	Applied the nappy, dressed the baby and wrapped up warmly				
16.	Rinsed well and cleaned with soapy water and dried				
17.	Washed and dried hands				
18.	Documented and reported any abnormal findings				

Signature of Student--

Signature of Clinical Instructor -------------------------------

Performance Evaluation: Breastfeeding

Definition

Breastfeeding is the best and most natural way of feeding a baby.

Purpose

1. To make sure breastfeeding is initiated soon after delivery.
2. To make sure breastfeeding is maintained as long possible, (ideally up to two years).
3. To make sure breastfeeding is established.
4. To make sure the mother is helped and advised on some of the problems of breastfeeding e.g. engorged breasts, sore nipples etc.
5. To make sure breastfeeding is on demand.
6. To make the mother understand the benefits of BF.
7. To promote bonding
8. To discourage artificial feeding to avoid infection.

Advatages of Breastfeeding

1. Breastfeeding develops a loving relationship between the mother and baby (bonding).
2. Breast milk gives the baby all the nourishment required.
3. Breast milk contains antibodies to protect the baby against infections and also protects the baby from allergic reactions.
4. Breast milk is the most hygienic and cleanest milk.
5. Breast milk is very cheap, it does not cost money.
6. Breast milk has easily digested proteins, lactose or milk sugar and fats.
7. Breastfeeding helps the woman regain her figure and health quickly i.e. causes the uterus to contract, which prevents prolonged blood loss. The pelvic muscles regain their tone quicker. The extra weight put on during pregnancy is used up in breastfeed.

Procedure

Sl. No.	Performance Criteria	S	U	NP	Comments
	Assessment				
1.	Ensured privacy				
2.	Assisted mother to change baby's nappy before starting feeding (if necessary)				
3.	Washed and dried hands (both nurse/ midwife and mother)				
4.	Ensured mother is comfortable before starting feeds, e.g. good posture, sitting or lying with back supported well and encouraged mother to empty her bladder				

Contd...

Contd...

Sl. No.	Performance Criteria	S	U	NP	Comments
5.	Exposed only one breast at a time				
6.	Mother is encouraged to position the baby close to her breast				
7.	Assisted the mother to start feeds on alternate breast each time				
8.	Helped the baby to Burp by putting him upright on Mum's (Nurse's) shoulders				
9.	Gently rubbed baby's back each time is removed from the breast				
10.	After completion of feeding, wrapped the baby properly and settle in his cot lying him on his side				
11.	Encouraged the mother to wipe nipple and areola with damp tissue and dry thoroughly				
12.	Applied breast pads and well fitting brassiere, if available				
13.	Left the mother comfortable				
14.	Washed hands after procedure				
15.	Documented appropriately and report any abnormal finding				

Signature of Student---

Signature of Clinical Instructor -------------------------------

Performance Evaluation: Eye Care of the Newborn

Introduction

Routine eye care is taken while bathing the baby, but special care is taken only when the presence of a discharge is noted. Therefore, if only one eye is infected, just that one to be taken care without touching other eye.

Eye care should be performed if discharge is present,. prior to breast-feeding to prevent spread of infection to the mother's breast.

Eye care is carried out before the application of any prescribed eye drops or ointment.

A swab should be taken if the infant has a discharge from the eyes.

Equipment

Sterile swab and transport medium

Pathology request completed and signed by the doctor.

Procedure

1. To be performed prior to eye care.
2. Remove swab from the tube. Ensure that stick or cotton bud end of swab is not touched.

3. Wipe cotton bud across eye from inner to outer corner ensuring discharge is collected in the swab.
4. Put swab into capped transport medium. Label it and send to microbiology with completed request form.

Care of Eyes

Equipment

1. 2 x 5 mL ampoules of sterile water
2. Sterile cotton wool balls
3. Disposal bag

Procedure

Sl. No.	Performance Criteria	S	U	NP	Comments
	Assessment				
1.	Carried out eye care as part of the baby's routine care				
2.	Explained to the baby's parents about the procedure				
3.	Washed hands and open pack on clean surface				
4.	Opened the ampoules and sterile cotton wool ready for use				
5.	Ensured that an eye swab has been taken prior to commencement of treatment				
6.	Started cleaning first with the less effected eye				
7.	Squeezed some sterile water on to the cotton wool ball. Clean the eye from the bridge of the nose outward using the cotton wool ball once only then discarded it				
8.	Repeated (if necessary) using one swab for each wipe				
9.	Dried the eye in the same manner				
10.	Applied topical treatment as prescribed (always attend the less affected eye first then more affected one)				
11.	Discarded the soiled swabs in the appropriate container away from working surface and washed and dried hands				
12.	Recorded in nursing notes that eye care is carried out. Including the description of the discharge or condition of the eye				

Signature of Student---

Signature of Clinical Instructor ------------------------------

Note:

1. Use one bottle for both eyes as long as it does not come directly into contact with eye.

2. Check with another nurse before instilling the drops.
3. Use 4th hourly or 6th hourly as prescribed and continue for 48 hours after symptom disappears.
4. Remaining drug will be stored for next use (for the same baby) as per the hospital policy.

Performance Evaluation: Gastric Lavage-Neonatal

Definition

Gastric lavage is the process of washing out stomach cavity by using water. Gastric lavage may be done to remove meconium, liquor, or mucus following delivery.

Purpose

1. To prevent vomiting and encourage feeding.
2. To aid absorption during feeding.
3. To prevent meconium irritation and aspiration (in case of meconium present in the stomach).

Procedure

Sl. No.	Performance Criteria	S	U	NP	Comments
	Assessment				
1.	Identified the baby and explain the procedure to the mother				
2.	Washed and dried hands.				
3.	Assembled equipment and wrapped baby well. To immobilize, laid the baby on right side				
4.	Estimated length of tube to be passed (xiphisternum to bridge of nose to ear)				
5.	Gently passed tube through nostril to stomach to the pre measured length				
6.	Aspirated stomach contents using 2 or 5 mL syringe, and placed on litmus paper to confirm position of tube				
7.	Secured the tube in place and send the fluid to lab for culture and sensitivity (if required)				
8.	Attached 10 mL syringe barrow to Nasogastric tube and poured water into syringe. Allow water to flow by gravity				
9.	Removed the syringe barrow and re-attach 5 mL syringe, aspirated the water gently. Confirmed that amount aspirated should equal to amount introduced				

Contd...

Contd...

Sl. No.	Performance Criteria	S	U	NP	Comments
10.	Identified amount of water used depends on size of baby. (Less than 2 kg use 15 mL, over 2 kg, use 20 mL)				
11.	Repeated the procedure until water is clear				
12.	Removed nasogastric tube after procedure, to be kept in position if it required further				
13.	Washed hands after procedure. Cleared trolley and stored equipment appropriately after washing and drying				
14.	Documented appropriately and reported any abnormal finding				

Signature of Student--

Signature of Clinical Instructor -------------------------------

Performance Evaluation: Heel Prick Blood Collection

Purpose

To ensure that correct technique is employed so as to prevent any serious complications, or the necessity of repeating procedure due to poor technique.

1. Heel puncture is performed on infants who require the following tests like blood glucose monitoring, capillary blood gas sampling, serum bilirubin test etc.
2. Before performing a heel puncture for any reason, the Nurse should ensure that the doctor is not performing a venipuncture in the near future so that unnecessary puncturing and handling of the baby can be avoided.

Equipment

1. Lancet or equivalent
2. Alcohol swab
3. Sterile cotton wool balls
4. Hemoglucotest strip/Capillary tube
5. Reflolux machine/Glucometer

Procedure

Sl. No.	Performance Criteria	S	U	NP	Comments
	Assessment				
1.	Washed and dried hands thoroughly				
2.	Chosen the site for puncture. (alternate heels and sides of feet)				

Contd...

Contd...

Sl. No.	Performance Criteria	S	U	NP	Comments
3.	Cleaned the selected site with alcohol swab and wiped dry with cotton wool ball				
4.	Circled heel with thumb and first finger and applied gentle pressure to produce a degree of engorgement. (If the heel is not well perfused, rub it or warm it with gauze soaked in warm water)				
5.	Punctured heel with lancet and accumulated a large drop of blood using gentle pressure				
6.	Allowed blood to fall directly onto the test strip area. (The blood must be sufficient to cover it completely). Followed the instructions for the appropriate glucometer				
7.	Applied gentle but firm pressure to the puncture site with a sterile cotton wool ball				
8.	Alternatively collected blood in a capillary tube by occluding one end of the tube with a finger tip and placing the open end of tube on the puncture site where blood has collected (This will provide a vacuum to allow blood to collect in the capillary tube)				
9.	Washed and dried hands				
10.	Ensured the baby is comfortable and checked the puncture site again				
11.	Documented appropriately				

Signature of Student---

Signature of Clinical Instructor --------------------------------

Complications of Poor Technique

1. Osteomylitis can occur due to poor technique and frequent puncturing of the calcaneous, resulting in chondritis. This can lead to long-term problems, including painful walking in later years.
2. Severe bruising due to excessive pressure being applied and faulty holding technique.
3. Scarring may also result in a degree of tenderness.

Performance Evaluation: Hypothermia Prevention of Neonatal

Purpose

To maintain warmth in the neonate and to prevent neonatal heat loss.

Policy

Caution must be taken to prevent the mechanism of neonatal heat loss through conduction, convection, radiation and evaporation.

Refrain from bathing the newborn immediately post delivery, until stabilization of temperature is within normal range.

When bathing a neonate wash and dry only a small area of the body at a time, keeping the rest of the infant's body covered.

Procedure

Care given in the delivery room:

Procedure

Sl. No.	Performance Criteria	S	U	NP	Comments
	Assessment				
1.	Dried the baby well and wrapped with a sterile warm dry towel following cutting of the umbilical cord				
2.	Placed the baby in a prewarmed incubator				
3.	Dressed the baby with baby cloths and wrapped appropriately with a warm dry towel and blankets, covering the head				
4.	Checked the baby's temperature at birth and before transportation to a postnatal ward				
5.	Kept the baby warm under a heater, until the body temperature is maintained prior to transfer				
6.	**Subsequent care in a postnatal ward.** Maintained the environmental temperature of the postnatal ward adequately warm to provide infants with adequate protection from convective heat loss. At all times by appropriate wrapping.				
7.	Checked the infant's temperature is below 37° centigrade, wrapped with extra blankets and placed infant in a cot with a vented plastic (Flexi glass) shield (Note If the infant is preterm, nurse in a pre-warmed incubator)				
8.	Avoided unnecessary exposure when attending to baby's needs.				
9.	Monitored the baby's temperature (according to policy and procedure) at hourly intervals until temperature has been stabilized at the normal range, i.e. 36.8 to 37 Centigrade.				
10.	Documented appropriately				

Signature of Student---

Signature of Clinical Instructor -------------------------------

Performance Evaluation: Incubator: Transferring/Changing

Purpose

To provide guidelines concerning the timing and reasons for transferring/changing an incubator.

Policy

1. Two nurses are required to perform this procedure safely.
2. Incubators will routinely changed on a weekly basis during the night shift (at early morning hour) unless contraindicated by the baby's condition.
3. If a child requires barrier or reverse barrier nursing.
4. If the incubator is very soiled and hence a potential source of infection.
5. If there is a mechanical fault in the incubator.

Equipment

1. A clean and pre-heated incubator set to the baby's neutral thermal environmental temperature.
2. If the baby is ventilated then use either a large metal trolley or weight scales covered with a blanket or sheet plus an ambu bag and oxygen cylinder, and 2 nurses.
3. Incubator
4. Dressing trolley
5. Weight scales
6. Blanket/Sheet
7. Ambu resuscitator
8. Oxygen cylinder- 1

Procedure

Sl. No.	Performance Criteria	S	U	NP	Comments
	Assessment				
1.	Assessed baby's condition- color, respiration, apex, transcutaneous pulse oximetry, temperature, tolerance to handling, etc. (If the baby is too ill or unstable to tolerate the procedure, do not continue)				
2.	Explained the procedure to them and asked them to wait outside until the procedure is completed				
3.	Switched on incubator and preheat to baby's neutral thermal environmental temperature. Transferred the baby's personal equipment to the clean incubator				

Contd...

Contd...

Sl. No.	Performance Criteria	S	U	NP	Comments
4.	Removed excess equipment, e.g. dynamap cable, etc. (it is not necessary to disconnect the ECG leads)				
5.	Ensured that there is an adequate length of IV and arterial line tubing to reach to the trolley/scales before moving the infant				
6.	The first nurse transferred the baby to the trolley/ scales, covers with a wrap, bags and masks (hand ventilate) the baby at the same rate that he/she was being ventilated				
7.	Same time the second nurse removed the dirty incubator and plugs in the clean one in its place. Ensured power is switched on (If infant is not ventilated then transfer directly to the clean pre-warmed incubator)				
8.	Following transfer, observed infant for color, ventilation, etc.				
9.	Recorded incubator change date on the care plan				
10.	Transferred dirty incubator to the dirty utility room for thorough cleaning				
11.	Documented as per hospital policy				

Signature of Student--

Signature of Clinical Instructor ------------------------------

Performance Evaluation: Low Birth Weight Infant Care of

Definition

Infant weighing less than 2.5 kg

Purpose

1. To monitor adaptation to extrauterine life.
2. To optimize growth and development.
3. To prevent complications of low birth weight, e.g. hypothermia, hypoglycemia .
4. To promote establishment of breastfeeding.
5. To provide support for the parents.

Equipment

1. Thermometer
2. Stethoscope

3. Infant warmer, cot and linen
4. Warm clothing
5. Stockinette for hat, bootees and mittens
6. Reflocheck machine and test stripes
7. Breast milk
8. Weighing scales
9. Infant documentation

Procedure

Sl. No.	Performance Criteria	S	U	NP	Comments
	Assessment				
1.	Washed and dried hands and followed universal precautions				
2.	Obtained pertinent information in mother's history, relating to infant				
3.	Received infant into appropriate prepared cot				
4.	Ensured the infant is placed in an appropriate position under an infant warmer, dried and wrapped in a warm towel				
5.	Assessed general condition, color, muscle tone, activity and behavior. Observed for jitteriness and signs of hypoglycemia				
6.	Recorded temperature, respiration, apex beat and infant weight as per hospital policy				
7.	Checked cord clamp is secured and followed cord care as per hospital policy				
8.	Ensured correct identification name bands are in place as per hospital policy				
9.	Dressed the infant in warm clothing and placed under the infant warmer until maintaining own body temperature				
10.	Recorded the blood glucose level as per hospital policy				
11.	Put the baby to mother's breast within the first hour of birth. Followed on feeds as per hospital policy and Baby Friendly Hospital Initiative Policy				
12.	Recorded output of urine and stools noting color				
13.	Ensured the sister incharge is informed of the infant's condition and progress				
14.	Ensured parents are regularly informed of infant's progress and undertake all infant's condition and progress				
15.	Documented appropriately				

Signature of Student---

Signature of Clinical Instructor ------------------------------

Performance Evaluation: Newborn Baby Routine Care of

Definition

Care and observations of the newborn baby

Purpose

1. To ensure the well-being of the newborn.
2. To detect any abnormality.
3. To assist the mother in caring for her baby.

Equipment

1. Weighing scale, thermometer

Procedure

Sl. No.	Performance Criteria	S	U	NP	Comments
	Assessment				
1.	At the time of bathing carried out the daily examination of the baby				
2.	Washed and dried hands				
3.	Checked the presence of identity bands				
4.	The mother is encouraged to observe and participate in the procedure				
5.	Observed the baby's color noted sign of cyanosis, jaundice				
6.	Noted the respiration's				
7.	Observed the muscle tone				
8.	Checked the babies skin, especially in the folds and creases				
9.	Checked the babies weight				
10.	Checked the temperature				
11.	Asked the mother about the baby's bladder and bowel movement				
12.	Checked the umbilical cord to ensure its clean and dry				
13.	Checked the eyes , nose, ears and mouth				
14.	Observed the baby is breast fed with the proper position				

Contd...

Contd...

Sl. No.	Performance Criteria	S	U	NP	Comments
15.	Answered all questions of the mother regarding her baby				
16.	Documented pertinent information				
17.	Reported findings to nurse incharge				

Signature of Student--

Signature of Clinical Instructor --------------------------------

Performance Evaluation: Phototherapy in the Postnatal Ward

Definition

Phototherapy is a treatment which provides an alternative way of dealing with bilirubin in the blood when the liver is unable to conjugate the quantities produced.

Purpose

1. To care an infant receiving phototherapy.
2. When the serum bilirubin rises above the recommended levels for the neonate.
3. Phototherapy will be started prophylactically when an infant appears very jaundiced and results are pending.

Equipment

Phototherapy unit of the appropriate safety standard cot/incubator.
Eye protection essential to prevent retinal damage.

Procedure

Sl. No.	Performance Criteria	S	U	NP	Comments
	Assessment				
1.	Assembled equipment				
2.	Explained the parents about the procedure				
3.	Washed and dried hands				
4.	Undressed baby				
5.	Covered eyes				

Contd...

Contd...

Sl. No.	Performance Criteria	S	U	NP	Comments
6.	Turned on lamp keeping it at a height of 45 cm (or 18 inches) from the surface of the mattress.				
7.	Turned the baby regularly (at least 3–4 hourly) to coincide with nursing care in single/double phototherapy				
8.	Checked baby's temperature 4th hourly				
9.	Colleted blood for serum bilirubin levels (SBR) in every morning and as necessary and recorded in nursing progress sheet				
10.	Phototherapy is discontinued as per SBR reached the required level, and as per doctor's order				
11.	Documented appropriately				

Signature of Student--

Signature of Clinical Instructor -------------------------------

Nursing Points/Complications to Watch for

1. Hypothermia or Hyperthermia
2. Dehydration: Fluid intake should be increased by 3 hourly breast feeds or more frequent breastfeeding.
3. Eye care: The infant may develop conjunctivitis or retinal damage.
4. Loose stools due to increased gut motility- excoriation of buttocks.
5. Skin rashes/burns.

Performance Evaluation: Radiant Warmer Use of

Definition

The provision of an effective method of preventing or correcting hypothermia.

Purpose

To maintain the body temperature within an acceptable normal range.

Equipment

1. Radiant warmer
2. Thermometer
3. Frequent observation chart

Procedure

Sl. No.	Performance Criteria	S	U	NP	Comments
	Assessment				
1.	Checked that the equipment is clean and in working order				
2.	Explained the procedure to the parents				
3.	Positioned the warmer unit so that the heater is directly over the body of the baby				
4.	Kept the height of the heater at 2 feet above the body of the baby				
5.	Switched on the heater				
6.	Adjusted the heat control knob to maximum and checked that the heater warms up				
7.	Documented the baby's temperature hourly on the frequent observation chart				
8.	Adjusted the heat control knob according to the baby's temperature				
9.	Documented appropriately				

Signature of Student---

Signature of Clinical Instructor ------------------------------

Performance Evaluation: Sterilization of Feeding Utensils

Definition

Method of destroying bacteria by heat or chemical agents.

Purpose

To destroy bacteria and aid prevention of gastrointestinal infection.

Requirement

1. Infant feeding bottle with teat and cover
2. Bottle brush
3. Large pan with lid or large plastic container with lid – approx. 4–5 liter
4. Sterilizing agent
5. Stove or gas cooker

Procedure

Sl. No.	Performance Criteria	S	U	NP	Comments
	Assessment				
1.	Washed and dried hands				
2.	Washed bottle, teat and cover in hot soapy water using the bottle brush to remove all milk curds from base and neck of the bottle. Squeezed and rolled teat between finger and thumb to remove all curds				
3.	Rinsed the bottle, teat and cover in clean water. Ensured all soap has been removed				
4.	Placed the clean bottle, teat and cover in the pan which has clean boiling water				
5.	Boiled for 10 minutes, with lid on				
6.	Removed pan from heat and allowed to cool				
7.	Washed hands				
8.	Removed bottle, teat and cover, and proceed to make up the feed				
	Chemical Method				
9.	Washed the plastic container as for bottles and rinse all soap suds off				
10.	Followed manufacture's instructions to make up sterilizing solution				
11.	Immersed the bottle teats, covers and discs completely in solution, ensuring no air bubbles are present				
12.	Placed "float" over items and ensured all items are submerged. Covered the container with a well fitting lid				
13.	Left the items in the solution until sterilized, according to manufacturer's instructions				
14.	Washed and dried hands and removed items required when ready to make up feeds. (Do not rinse any of the sterilized items)				
15.	Changed the solution every 24 hours. Mark on container date and time when changed				

Signature of Student---

Signature of Clinical Instructor ------------------------------

Performance Evaluation: Transfer Incubator/Cot

Purpose

To provide guidelines for transfer from incubator to cot

Policy

1. Once the baby's general condition is stable, weight over 1.4 kg and maintaining own thermo-regulation.
2. Cots are changed routinely on a weekly basis. They will be changed more frequently if required.
3. Babies requiring a triple phototherapy will be nursed in cots.

Equipment

1. A clean cot
2. Clean linen

Procedure

Sl. No.	Performance Criteria	S	U	NP	Comments
	Assessment				
1.	Assessed the baby's general condition prior to transferring to a cot				
2.	Dressed the baby with warm linen, gown, mittens and booties and wrap in a blanket				
3.	Checked the baby's axilla temperature one hour after transferring into the cot (If temperature is less than 36.5°C use a heat shield)				
4.	Ensured that the cot is placed in a proper area				
5.	Checked auxillary temperature one hour later (If baby is hypothermic—use heat shield plus another blanket)				
6.	Rechecked temperature again one hour later. If still low, noted sister-incharge and prepared to transfer baby back into an incubator				
7.	Recorded on care plan the date of changing the cot.				
8.	Transferred dirty incubator/cot to dirty utility room for terminal cleaning				
	Cleaning of Cots				
10.	Wiped the insides of bassinet and cot flaps with plain water at every care time and dry thoroughly				

Contd...

Contd...

Sl. No.	Performance Criteria	S	U	NP	Comments
11.	After use, cleaned bassinet, mattress, cot frame and cupboards inside and out with soap and water. Avoided immersing mattress into water. Dried all equipments thoroughly. Damage/tear in mattress reported to sister incharge.				
12.	Re- stocked 1 sheet and 2 blankets. In cupboard – admission basket containing nappies, disposable bags, soap and dish, thermometer, shampoo, measuring tape, metal bowl. placed in appropriate area				
13.	Reported pertinent information to charge nurse				

Signature of Student--

Signature of Clinical Instructor -------------------------------

Performance Evaluation: Umbilical Cord Care

Definition

The care and management of infants who have a malodorous/inflamed/infected umbilical cord.

Normally, an uninfected cord should be cleaned to prevent signs of infection.

Purpose

1. To inspect the umbilical cord in each nappy change.
2. To take a swab for culture and sensitivity prior to the initial cleaning.
3. To perform care only when there is inflammtion/infection or smell from the umbilical cord.

Equipment

1. Several alcohol swabs.
2. Cord Clamp cutters'

Procedure

Sl. No.	Performance Criteria	S	U	NP	Comments
	Assessment				
1.	Washed and dried hands				
2.	Removed cord clamps 48 hours after initial application. Observed cord is dry and necrosed, by cutting through the hinge of the clamp				

Contd...

Contd...

Sl. No.	Performance Criteria	S	U	NP	Comments
3.	Cleaned surrounding area of cord with alcohol swabs applying particular attention to the space between the cord and the skin				
4.	Folded nappy away from umbilical stump				
5.	Disposed of dirty items				
6.	Recorded condition of cord stump on infant's chart, and reported to sister incharge				

Signature of Student--

Signature of Clinical Instructor --------------------------------

Important Points to Remember

1. Umbilical cord care will be performed if there is bleeding or signs of infection such as redness, odor or discharge.
2. If any purulent discharge is obvious at the cord site, notify the doctor and take a swab for culture and sensitivity. Record on care plan.
3. Antiseptic powder or ointment should not be applied (unless medically indicated) to the umbilical stump, neither should dressings. It should be left open and uncovered.
4. The umbilical cord will dry out and usually fall off during the first 7–10 days of life. If this does not occur, be alert for signs of insidious infection.

CHAPTER

19

General Performance Evaluation

Criteria for Clinical Diary Evaluation

Students are required to write daily diary of their clinical experience.
Student should write minimum 2 patients detail as follow.
Diary should include:

1. Date
2. Name of the ward
3. Number of patient in the ward
4. Name of the nurse incharge
5. Any critical patient in the ward/ number of critical patient in the ward
6. Number of nurses working in the unit
7. Name of the doctors (HOD)
8. Name of the patient
9. Date of admission
10. Diagnosis
11. Treatment received on time of admission
12. History of the patient (basic data, health history, family history in detail)
13. Physical examination at least students own assessment of physical examination of vital signs, any significant findings in the physical examination
14. One patient complete detail of lab value
15. One patient complete detail of drugs used
16. One patient care provided by the student
17. Write 5 terminology
18. Other assignment done by the student
19. New learning

Signature of Clinical Instructor **Signature of the Student**

Evaluation Performa for Teaching Practice

Name of the student teacher --Date --------

Level of students--Time -----------------

Topic --Evaluator ---------

Sl. No.	Criteria	Excellent	Good	Average	Satisfactory	Poor
1.	**Preparation** Classroom preparation appropriate					
2.	**Objectives** Clear, adequate, appropriate					
3.	**Introduction** Relevant					
4.	**Motivating**					
5.	**Subject matter** Relevant/adequate					
6.	Through knowledge about the topic					
7.	Explanation/ interpretation of the content					
8.	Adequacy and coverage of content					
9.	**Language** Correct use of terms and grammar					
10.	**Non-verbal communication** relevant and effective					
11.	**Audiovisual** Appropriate					
12.	Legible					
13.	Good use of blackboard					
14.	**Voice** Clear, audible, easy to follow					
15.	Modulation of voice					

Contd... .

Contd...

Sl. No.	Criteria	Excellent	Good	Average	Satisfactory	Poor
16.	**Personal attitude** Dress and posture/ well dressed					
17.	Good posture /cheerful and pleasant					
18.	Questioning technique					
19.	Students interaction/ clears doubts of the students					
20.	**Bibliography**					
	Total marks					

Remarks---

Signature of Evaluator -------------

Signature of Students ------------- Signature of Principal -------------

Scoring:

Excellent =5 (80–100)
Good = 4 (60–79)
Average = 39 (50–59)
Satisfactory = 2 (40–49)
Poor = 1 (below 39)

Evaluation Performa for Clinical Demonstration

Name of the Student ---------------------------------------Date ---------------

Name of the Procedures --

Sl. No.	Criteria	0	1	2	3	4
1.	**Planning**					
1.1.	Formulation of clear/appropriate objectives					
1.2.	Organization of content for procedure					
1.3.	Submission of plan in time					
2.	**Implementation**					
2.1.	Explanation and getting consent from the patient					
2.2.	Preparation of the unit and patient					
2.3.	Assembly of articles					
2.4.	Maintaining privacy and safety of the patient					
2.5.	Observation of the scientific principles					
2.6.	Adequate skill in performing procedure					
2.7.	Use of resources					
2.8.	Completeness of procedures					
3.	**Evaluation of post-procedure responsibilities**					
3.1.	Achievement of the objectives					
3.2.	Comforting the patient					
3.3.	Replacement of articles					
3.4.	Recording and reporting					
	Total marks					

Signature of Student---------------------------

Signature of the Evaluator--

Score

Excellent = 4
Good = 3
Average = 2
Satisfactory = 1
Poor = 0

Conference Evaluation Form

These are free suggestions for questions about conference evaluation. These conference survey evaluation items are designed for attendees to answer, not presentors, they are presented as survey design samples only. The questions are provided as possible example of type of questions you might want to include.

Participants Information

Please note your profession and status	• GNM • B.Sc. Nursing • PBBS.C Nursing • MSc. Nursing • Administrator • University faculty
Please note years in your profession	

Please tell us how satisfied you were with the following?

1. How satisfied were you with the registration process?
   - Very dissatisfied
   - Dissatisfied
   - Satisfied
   - Very satisfied
2. How satisfied were you with the conference material provided?
   - Very dissatisfied
   - Dissatisfied
   - Satisfied
   - Very satisfied
3. Overall, how satisfied were you with the speakers/presenters?
   - Very dissatisfied
   - Dissatisfied
   - Satisfied
   - Very satisfied
4. Overall, how satisfied were you with the conference facilities?
   - Very dissatisfied
   - Dissatisfied
   - Satisfied
   - Very satisfied
5. How many sessions did you attended?
6. Did you feel the length of the conference session were too long just about right or too short?
   - Too long
   - Just about right
   - Too short

7. The content of the conference session was appropriate and informative.
    - Strongly disagree
    - Disagree
    - Agree
    - Strongly agree
8. The conference was well-organized.
    - Strongly disagree
    - Disagree
    - Agree
    - Strongly agree
9. Conference staff was helpful and courteous.
    - Strongly disagree
    - Disagree
    - Agree
    - Strongly agree
10. What kinds of sessions would you like to see included at future conference?
    - Strongly disagree
    - Disagree
    - Agree
    - Strongly agree

Please help us make this conference better next year by filling out this short questionnaire. You may turn in your questionnaire at the registration desk when you leave, or mail it to------------------

Sl. No.	Criteria	Very satisfied	Satisfied	Dissatisfied	Very dissatisfy
1.	Please rate your overall satisfaction with the conference				
2.	Please rate your overall satisfaction with the exhibits area				
3.	Please rate your overall satisfaction with the format of the conference (i.e. morning sessions, breaks, lunch, afternoon session/ breakout)				
4.	Please rate your overall satisfaction with the reception and breaks				

Contd...

Contd...

Sl. No.	Criteria	Very satisfied	Satisfied	Dissatisfied	Very dissatisfy
5.	Please rate your overall satisfaction with the facilities				
6.	Please rate your overall satisfaction with the location of the conference				
7.	Overall, based on your total experience at the conference, will you attend or recommend someone else attend next conference				
8.	Please provide any comments you have on future conference, locations, topics, speakers. Or general suggestions regarding the conference				

Workshop Evaluation Form

Sl. No.	Criteria	Strongly disagree 1	Disagree 2	Agree 3	Strongly disagree 4
1.	The program objectives were met				
2.	Accuracy and utility of content were discussed				
3.	Content was appropriate				
4.	Teaching methods were effective				
5.	Visual aids, hand outs, and oral presentations clarified content				
	Presenter 1				
6.	Knew the subject matter				
7.	Taught the subject completely				
8.	Presented content in an organized manner				
9.	Maintained the interest of participants				
10.	Answered questions effectively				
	Presenter 2				
6.	Knew the subject matter				
7.	Taught the subject completely				
8.	Presented content in an organized manner				
9.	Maintained the interest of participants				
10.	Answered questions effectively				
	Presenter 3				

Professional and Ethical Issues

Sl. No.	Criteria	Strongly disagree 1	Disagree 2	Agree 3	Strongly disagree 4
	Professional ethical issue				
1.	Facility was adequate				
2.	Special needs were met				
3.	Facility was comfortable and accessible				

Contd...

Contd...

Sl. No.	Criteria	Strongly disagree 1	Disagree 2	Agree 3	Strongly disagree 4
4.	Food and beverage were adequate (if applicable)				
5.	Information could be applied to my practice (if applicable)				
6.	Information could contribute to achieving personal or professional goals				
7.	Did this program enhance your professional expertise				

What was your overall impression of the activity/what went well/ what could have been improved?
What did you learn that was new or different? How will this information change how you practice?
What topics or presenters would you like to see at future?
Other comments

Lesson Plan

What is a Lesson Plan

A lesson plan "is actually a plan of action" (lesser B Sands). A lesson plan reveals knowledge and philosophy of the teacher, her/his understanding of students, objectives of education, the content to be taught and teaching ability to utilize appropriate methods of teaching, it points out what has been taught and in what direction the student must be guided.

It is the teacher's mental and emotional visualization of the classroom experiences as he plans it to occur. It is the core of effective teaching, it is the blue print of what a teacher is going to do.

There should be bold heading and small heading indicating the different things that occur at different times. Who are to do those things Teacher and students activities. The subject matter to be taught and methods to teach. It begins with goals or objectives of instruction and ends with means to arrive at those goals. Finally a method to evaluate whether it set goals have been achieved.

Why Lesson Planning (Purpose)

1. It focuses on consideration of goals and objectives, selection of subject matter, selection of procedure, the planning of activities and the preparation of test of progress, thus it guides the teacher in presentation of subject matter and activities involved.
2. It keeps the teacher on the tracks; ensure steady progress and a definite outcome of teaching and learning procedure.
3. It is essential for effective teaching.
4. It prevents waste of time-help teacher to be systematic and orderly, it encourages organization of subject matter and activities and prevent haphazard teaching and minimizing chance of omitting some vital part of the lesson.
5. It helps the teacher to delimit the teaching field.
6. It encourages proper consideration of the learning process and the choice of appropriate learning procedures and employs the best technique, to judge the outcome of instruction.
7. It serves as a check on unplanned curriculum—continuity and inter-connectedness can be planned and at the same time avoid repetition.
8. Planning encourages the teacher to consider the need and level of understanding of students.
9. Lesson planning gives the teacher greater confidence and greater freedom in teaching.

Points to Remember in Planning a Lesson Plan

- The lesson plan should contain only main points/ideas or concepts. It is not necessary to write down every word a teacher is going to say which means the teacher will only read out the material and not teach or explain the matter
- A teacher may use her own subject notes which is different from the lesson plan
- The teacher should not become over dependent on the lesson plan. The plan must be flexible, not rigid and adjusted according to the situation arising in the classroom
- A fresh plan should be prepared every time a teacher takes a class that the subject matter does not become redundant
- Design for sequencing the subject matter. The design may be either to present the subject matter by giving main heading and subheading etc. or it can also be by developing a concept, comparision or problem solving designs
- Planning must be done keeping in mind the level of understanding of the students and their previous experiences
- The method of teaching planned must be according to the subject to be attained cognitive, affective, or psychomotor skill development
- Certain psychological factors related to learning should also be remembered when planning a lesson. Organization of the content must be logical and meaningful and the sequence should progress from simple to complex, from concrete to abstract and plan to known to unknown
- Motivation to maintain interest and attention of the class is important while planning and presenting subject matter
- Each lesson is planned in such a way that the objective of each lesson lead to the attainment of unit objectives than course objective and finally the objective of the curriculum.

Pre-requisites for Good Lesson Plan

- The teacher must have adequate mastery over subject matter and practice if it is for skill lesson
- The teacher must understand the student's traits, interest and background, social cultural in order to make a plan of teaching suitable for them
- The teacher must be fully conversant with new methods and technique of teaching her/his subject
- Teacher must have a good understanding of psychology of learning, philosophy of education, sociology and educational psychology and culture of the community
- Ensure active learner participation during a class and maintain interest and motivation of student. Avoid boredom
- There should be variety and novelty in type of presentation.

Essential Elements of Good Lesson Plan

The plan should state clearly the outcomes to be achieved including both central and contributory objectives. The contributory objectives.

1. Topic
2. Group
3. Place
4. Method of teaching
5. Medium of instruction
6. Teaching aids
7. Name of the student teacher
8. Background of the students
9. Numbers of students
10. Duration
11. Time

General Objectives: At the end of the program, the participants will be able to:

Lesson Plan Format

Sl. No.	Time	Specific objectives	Content	Teaching-learning activities	AV aids used	Evaluation

Preoperative Checklist

Preoperative Nursing Checklist

Health agency name----------------------------- Hospital No.-------------------------

Name of the patient-----------------------------Age --------------------------Ward------------------Bed No.----------Date----------------------Proposed operation --------------------------------Name of the surgeon---Consent signed: Yes/No

Height ---------------Weight------------------------Allergies--------------------------

Temperature----------------Pulse----------------------Respiration---------------------

Blood pressure-------------------Urine sugar %------------------Ketone --------------

Protein-----------------------Blood group-------------------FBS-------------------------

Identification band: Yes /No
Crown: Yes /No
Dentures removed: Yes/No
Glasses/lenses removed: Yes /No
Jewellery removed: Yes /No
Makeup/nail polish removed: Yes /No
Hairpin removed: Yes /No
Nasogastric tube in place: Yes /No
Bladder emptied: Yes /No
Catheter present: Yes /No
Theater gown: Yes /No
Skin preparation done: Yes /No
Premeditation-given: Yes/No. At---------------by--------------

Received in the theater Nurse Name--------------------

Performance Appraisal Report

Performance Appraisal

Name --Staff number--------------------

Designation ----------------------- Grade -----------------------Department ---------

Evaluation period -------------- To----------------------

Purpose

1. The purpose of this appraisal is to provide opportunity for the appraiser to discuss work performance with the appraise and find ways of improving the performance and increasing job satisfaction.
2. The rating of POOR will be reappraised in 3 months.

Tick as Appropriate

Rating	01 < than 55	02 (56–70)	03 (71–80)	04 (81–90)	05 (90–100)
	Poor	Average	Good	Very good	Excellent
1. Ability to express ideas and view points in a logical and systemic manner	Unable to express ideas	Express ideas not in a logical manner	Sometimes express logically	Mostly express ideas and viewpoint in logical systematic manner	Logical in presenting ideas
2. Flexibility and objectivity in accepecting new ideas and view points	Rigid	Rarely accepts others opinion or new ideas	Occasionally accepts others views and ideas	Mostly accepting	Always accepts new ideas and implements
3. Motivation to learn and promote professional skills	Doesn't show any interest	Rarely works At improving professional skills	Sometimes assist with staff development programs	Contributes regularly	Participates actively
4. Relationship with superior	Not communicating through proper channels	Not getting along with direct superior	Mostly getting along with superior	Always maintain good professional relationship	Highly efficient in maintaining relationship
5. Professionwise relations with colleagues	Never support or help colleagues	Rarely cooperate and help colleagues	Cooperative in general	Mostly cooperative and help initiative to assist colleagues	Has an excellent relationship with colleagues

Contd...

Contd...

Rating	01 < than 55	02 (56–70)	03 (71–80)	04 (81–90)	05 (90–100)
6. Conduct with clientele	Never responds clients problems	Rarely shows interest to find and solve clients problems	Has fairly good relationship to client	Pleasant disposition while interacting with clients	Appreciated by all clients
7. Reliability	Unreliable	Rarely reliable	Reliable at most time	Reliable to accomplish goals	Extremely competent and possess high sense of responsibility
8. Punctuality and adherence to working hours	Often absent	Frequently late	Usually present on time	Rarely absent or late	Always punctual
9. Knowledge of rules and procedures of works	Does not adheres to policies and procedures	Inadequate knowledge	Possess basic knowledge of rules and procedures	Complies standards of nursing practices	Highly knowledgeable and resourceful
10. Productivity (performance standards related to time)	Fails to complete assigned work	Limited performance	Generally meets the standards of time	Adhere establish time frame	Highly productive
11. Productivity (accuracy and proficiency)	Lacks proficiency in carrying out duties	Always needs guidance and correction	Occasionally needs guidance and correction	Works well needs source guidance in specialized areas	Highly efficient
12. Ability to plan and program his/her work	Unable to plan	Less organized need guidance	Organized on most cases, planning up to the standard	Well organized	Highly professionally organized
13. Ability to organize and coordinate work	Inability to organize	Minimum ability in organizing	Generally able to organize and coordinate	Demonstrate good organization most of the time	Actively involved in organizing distributing teaching and follow-up care
14. Ability to review work	Not up to the expectation	Shows ability with constant supervision	Fairly accurate requires minimal supervision	Accurate and able to meet job needs	Works independently and efficiently

Contd...

Contd...

Rating	01 < than 55	02 (56–70)	03 (71–80)	04 (81–90)	05 (90–100)
15. Ability to monitor and assess work	Unable to monitor assess the work of subordinate	Lacks adequate knowledge and ability to assess and monitor the work of subordinate	Occasionally needs assistance	Resourceful and capable of assessing and monitoring the subordinate	Always displays perfect with efficiency, possess leadership quality and competent
16. Ability to take appropriate decisions	Unable to take appropriate decisions	Needs guidance in taking appropriate decisions	Has basic capabilities , occasionally needs guidance and supervision	Take appropriate decision most of the time	Highly efficient and takes excellent decision at all circumstances
17. Ability to analyze and suggest appropriate solutions for work related problems	Does not possess ability to analyze and suggest solutions	Need help and guidance to analyze and suggest appropriate solution	Capable of accepting problems giving appropriate suggestions, occasionally needs guidance	Good in analyzing suggesting appropriate suggestion most of the time	Highly competent skilled in analyzing and suggesting appropriate decisions
18. Ability to work under pressure	Commits mistakes	Has difficulty in cooperating with work pressure	Has capability under pressure	Copes with work load in most cases	Manages crisis situation efficiently
19. Ability to prepare memorandums and reports	Unable to prepare memorandums and reports	Able to do with guidance	With little assistance able to prepare	Good in preparing memorandum and report	Independently prepares memorandum and report
20. Ability to take initiative and innovate proposal to promote system and procedures	Lack of initiative	Rarely initiative in promoting system	Generally initiative and shows interests	Takes on initiative to promote system	Highly initiative and successful in developing quality care

Give examples which show ability (positive factors) and others which show weakness (negative factors) especially in case where maximum and minimum rating have been given

----

Comments/recommendations --

On the basis of the above comments, the appraise is evaluated as:

Poor----- Average ---- Good----Very good--------Excellent

Appraisees comments (if any)

Appraisee's signature Appraisers
Signature

Date--------------------
Designation------------------

Date -------------------- Date------------------

Nursing Director/Officer's/Incharge signature ----------------------------

(Rating poor will be reappraised in 3 months / referred to staff development section)

Executive Jobs Performance Appraisal Report for Any Seniors jobs

1. Period covered by this report; from --------------------to--------------------
2. Name --
3. Nationality ---------------------------------------File No.------------------------
4. Date of birth---
5. Date of appointment--
6. Grade ---------------------------Class ---
7. Date occupying this grade --
8. Designation --
9. Academic qualifications:
10. List the last three academic certificates, commencing by the last obtained;

Title of certificate	Specialization	Year obtained	School/college/university

1. Attention to appearance :

Always attentive	Attentive at most time	Average attention	In attentive in many cases	Not attentive	Rating
5	4	3	2	1	

2. Acceptance of advice and guidance:

Always understanding and accepting	Understanding and accepting at most times	Average in accepting guidance	Not accepting guidance in most cases	Not accepting guidance nor advice	Rating
5	4	3	2	1	

3. Interest in the promotion and development of working methods and techniques:

Always interested	Interested in most cases	Average	Limited interest	Poor interest	Rating
5	4	3	2	1	

4. Relation with superiors:

Excellent	Good	Average	Below standard	Unsatisfactory	Rating
5	4	3	2	1	

5. Professionwise relations with colleagues:

Always cooperative	Mostly co-operative	Cooperative in general	Little interest to cooperate	Absolutely uncooperative	Rating
5	4	3	2	1	

6. Ability to determine and fulfill the needs of the public:

High	Good	Needs more guidance	Needs much guidance	Unsatisfactory	Rating
5	4	3	2	1	

7. Reliability:

Always reliable	Reliable at most times	Needs some guidance	Needs much guidance	Requires continuous guidance	

Degree of Efficiency

Factors of Assessment

8. Punctuality and adherence to working hours:

Always punctual and adherent	Punctual in most cases	Punctual in general	Punctual a certain extent	Often absent	Rating
5	4	3	2	1	

9. Knowledge of job duties and responsibilities:

Full knowledge	Good knowledge	Average	Ignores some duties	Limited knowledge	Rating
5	4	3	2	1	

10. Knowledge of rules, regulations and procedures of work:

Competent	Knowledgeable in general	Average	Below average	Limited knowledge	Rating

11. Technical knowledge of works systems and procedures:

Competent	Knowledgeable in general	Average	Below average	Limited knowledge	Rating
5	4	3	2	1	

12. Productivity (performance standards related to time):

Above standards	Within standards	Average	Below average	Poor	Rating
5	4	3	2	1	

13. Productivity (accuracy and proficiency):

Highly accurate and proficient	Good	Average	Below average	Poor	Rating
5	4	3	2	1	

14. Ability to work without continued supervision:

Does not need supervision	Rarely needs supervision	Sometime needs supervision	Mostly needs supervision	Always needs supervision	Rating
5	4	3	2	1	

15. Abreast of modern professional knowledge and skills:

Abreast	Abreast in most cases	Average	Rarely abreast	Not interested	Rating
5	4	3	2	1	

16. Skill in applying modern working methods and techniques:

Highly skilled	Skilled	Fair	Less than required	Poor skill	Rating
5	4	3	2	1	

17. Ability to work under pressure:

High capability and positive response	Good	Appropriate	Commits some mistakes	Negative response	Rating
5	4	3	2	1	

18. Ability to prepare messages and memorandums:

Excellent	Good	Average	Less than average	Poor	Rating
5	4	3	2	1	

19. Adherence to safety and prevention procedures (including files and technical equipments):

Always adherent	Adheres at most times	Average	Is not adherent at most times	Does not care	Rating
Grand total					

20. Ability to take initiative and provide suggestions to promote systems and procedures:

Always has initiative	Frequently has initiative	Sometime has initiative	Rarely has initiative	Has no initiative	Rating
5	4	3	2	1	
Grand total					

Please give examples which shows ability (positive factors) and others which show weakness (negative factors) especially in cases where maximum rating has been given

----

Grand Total

Excellent	from 90 to 100
Very good	from 80 to less than 90
Good	from 70 to less than 80
Satisfactory	from 55 to less than 70
Poor	less than 55

In light of above assessment, do you feel that:

- The qualifications and capabilities of this official do not qualify him to assume higher responsibilities
- This official has been placed in the proper position and grade suitable to his skills and abilities
- This official is efficient in his present duties and is capable to assume higher responsibilities.

Recommendations

In view of the positive and negative factors in the official personal capabilities and performance, please explain how the positive aspects could be strengthened and suggest ways to overcome the negative aspects, specifying the kind of training required if suggested:

Report prepared by: --Signature ------------------

Designation: --- Date -----------------------

Remarks by higher supervisors:

Name: --Signature -----------------------------

Designation: ---------------------------------Date ------------------------------------

Countersigned by head of the unit/institution

Signature --------------------------------------

Date --

General Guidelines for Completion of Evaluation Form

Supervisory Jobs

This group includes official who are occupying professional supervisory jobs. These working assignments are primarily related to assessment, planning and implementation according to the working system and regulations as well as assignment from their direct supervisors.

1. Basic information in this form should be completed according to records available in the official file.
2. The immediate supervisor(who prepares the report) would tick in the appropriate square. The number noted in the rating square.
3. The total number of rating should be scored in the specified square upon covering all factors.
4. Examples required to show the strong and weak points in the official performance, capabilities and behavior should depend on actual incidents that happened.

   Example 1

   An official scores maximum grade 5 in initiative and suggesting innovative proposal to promote systems and procedures. (For example, this official has prepared a systematic report to simplify systems and procedures in this department. When the recommendations stated in his report have been implemented, it resulted in simplification of procedures and consequently saved time and resources).

   Example 2

   An official obtained the minimum grade 1 in punctuality and adherence to working hours. This employee is absent for an average of 5days every month without any justified reason. Moreover, he is not adhering to the official working hours in most cases. He has been warned verbally and writing. Yet, he is not adhering to official working hours.
5. Where recommendations are required to strengthen the positive factors and overcome negative factors, please specify recommendations including training or any other system.
6. After countersigned the report by heads of the department any official who are rated poorly, should be notified in writing specifying to him his points of weakness so as to improve his performance.
7. The report should be filled in the official file. Recommendations and information contained therein should be utilized in all personnel aspects which arise within 1 year from the date of preparing the report.

Index

G

H

I

L

M

N

O

P